The Care Leader's Handbook

A practical guide to leadership for care managers, team leaders and future superstars.

Sophie and Rob Coulthard

Copyright 2019 Sophie and Rob Coulthard
All rights reserved.
ISBN: 978-1-09-392142-7

The Care Leader's Handbook
ISBN: 978-1-09-392142-7
Independently published through KDP. This is version 2.

Author's note: Some names in this work may have been changed.

Cover design: arslanubaid from fiverr.com
Illustrations and graphics: Daniel from Explainshow

Playlist: Endless chill-hop playlists on Spotify for Sophie, and a bit of Northern Soul and Ibiza classics for Rob

www.CareLeadersHandbook.co.uk – for all additional resources relating to the book.

www.JudgementIndex.co.uk
@JudgementIndex on Twitter, LinkedIn and Facebook
0800 8101025

For all enquiries including bulk orders and speaking or media, please contact: **gabby@judgementindex.co.uk**

Dedication

To all the incredible care professionals who make a difference in people's lives every day.

And to our families for putting up with us while we wrote this book!

Contents

About the authors
Our choice of language
Introduction

About the authors

ROB COULTHARD

Rob is an experienced leadership consultant, trainer and coach and has delivered analysis and training workshops for a variety of organisations around the world. He fulfilled all his military ambitions during his 26 years in the British Army having progressed from boy soldier to a commissioned officer.

In 2008 he was introduced to the Judgement Index and the concept of assessing values to predict performance and risk, for the benefit of individuals and teams. Rob now concentrates on facilitating dramatic changes in the organisations he works with, in staff retention, culture and quality of performance. He is a firm believer in generating responsibility at all levels, flexible charismatic leadership and good judgement.

Rob lives with his family in their old thatch cottage on Salisbury Plain and counts among his hobbies cooking, red wine and keeping the latter in check by physical training.

SOPHIE COULTHARD

Sophie is Rob's daughter, and having spent many school holidays sat at the back of Rob's lectures and workshops, she absorbed a lot of his leadership methods and strategies. All of this came in handy when at 21 she became the manager of a busy late-night bar, responsible for a large team of staff and doormen. This role became her crash course in leadership.

Moving into the corporate world and becoming a self-confessed "job-hopper", Sophie witnessed companies who weren't doing enough to develop their culture and values in order to retain staff, so after joining her dad full time at Judgement Index, she realised she could help companies make a difference and become great companies to work for.

She's also passionate about sharing best practice in care and launched The Road To Outstanding podcast in 2017. The podcast is focused on sharing experiences, stories and strategies from inspirational care managers and industry experts and to date has had over 10,000 downloads.

Sophie lives in South West London and enjoys exploring the city on her yellow bike and discovering hidden coffee shops.

Our choice of language

We wanted to keep the language we use throughout the book consistent, and as there are lots of different terms used across care, we decided, for simplicity to use the following:

Care Professionals – We debated a general term to cover people working in care, whether that be as a support or care worker, nurse, or something else. We refer to these people throughout the book as care professionals.

Company – Whether you work for a charity, social enterprise, a single care home or a large group; we will use the term "company" to describe any care organisation.

Home – when referring to a single location we will quite often use the term "home" but this can still apply to a domiciliary company where there may be a central office.

Leader – That's you! If you're reading this book then you are a leader, if of no one else then yourself. You may also be well into your leadership journey, a manager or area manager, a deputy, team leader or aspiring to any of those things.

Performance – We don't mean putting on a show! We simply mean how you perform when you're at work. Performing well is doing a good job.

Introduction

We've been working with care companies for quite a few years, either supporting them with their selection, staff and culture development and also running our successful leadership workshops and academies up and down the country.

We know that a leader's journey doesn't start and finish at the end of a course, so we wanted to produce a workbook to support our clients once they had finished a leadership academy with us. Originally, the plan was for it to be just that, a workbook, but recognising that there were not many books out there focusing on care leadership over management, our writing began.

It's common for companies to see an owner or CEO as a leader, the registered manager as a manager and everyone else as neither of these things, but regardless of role, every person has to fulfil a leader's role at times. This is why we called the book a leadership book. We will cross boundaries between leadership and management on occasion but please embrace our ethos of developing a leadership culture and you will get a lot from it, no matter what your level within your company.

We know that many care companies do not have the funding available to support their teams through leadership training or are not able to do as much of it as they would like. We wanted to create a book that could be accessible to anyone, with additional resources available online. Please head to the website to access these: **www.careleadershandbook.co.uk**

We were also inspired to write the book based on the many people who attend our courses and say that they wish they had learned this stuff years ago.

The book is separated into three sections: Leading Yourself, Leading Others and Leading The Culture, and we recommend reading the book all of the way through first, rather than diving into a specific section as the sections link together.

Part 1

Leading Yourself

Leadership starts with you

One question we always ask any group or audience is: "Who here is a leader?" and look to see how many raise their hand. We almost never see a full audience raise their hands to this question and from the start of this book we would like to change this mindset.

Everyone is a leader. You are a leader. If you're not the leader of anyone else, then at the very least you're the leader of yourself. Who gets you out of bed in the morning? Who leads those that you care for? Hopefully you're saying: "Me!" and that's what we want to encourage; self-leadership.

The world needs people to be leaders more than ever before. That doesn't necessarily mean more managers or CEO's, it just means people who can lead themselves and others when needed to a positive outcome.

The care sector also needs more leaders. A manager of a care company today has a greater workload than ever before, and so to have a team made up of confident self-leaders can make all the difference between a good care company and an exceptional one.

We believe that leaders are not born but developed through life's journey. Your own leadership skills have been developing since you were too small to know what leadership was, and no matter whether you're an experienced leader who's been on many courses or fresh into the sector, you will have picked up and honed your own leadership style over the years. Even the most experienced leaders should take the time to learn new techniques and reflect on their own performance.

Before we start the journey and share our favourite leadership strategies and techniques we are going to begin with a self-reflection and analysis of where you are right now.

Analysing yourself

Now that we've established that you are a leader, let's begin by analysing what your strengths are and what areas may need development. It's important to reflect every now and then at what you are good at and where there is room for improvement, and this will make a good starting point before you work your way through the book.

Have you ever done any analysis on your strengths and development areas? There are a number of ways you could have done this including:

- Survey staff for their opinion
- 360 feedback or appraisal
- Performance profiling or wheel (which you will see later in this book)
- Personality type tests
- Behavioural assessments or situational judgement tests
- Values-based assessments

If you've done any of these recently then you may already have some idea on where you stand. Write on the page opposite or download the template to print from the website: **www.careleadershandbook.co.uk** and ask yourself the following questions:

- What are my top 3 strengths as a leader?
- What are my biggest development areas?
- How would I describe my leadership style?
- How would my colleagues describe me as a leader? (be brave – ask someone who will give you an honest answer, and then others to get a full picture)

Hold on to this piece of paper and refer back to it as you work your way through the book. You'll learn more about your leadership style later and that may cause you to reflect on what you've originally written. The way your colleagues describe you may change too as you start to implement some of the techniques and strategies you'll learn.

MY TOP 3 STRENGTHS AS A LEADER ARE:

1. _____

2. _____

3. _____

MY DEVELOPMENT AREAS ARE:

_____

_____

_____

MY LEADERSHIP STYLES ARE:

_____

_____

_____

MY COLLEAGUES DESCRIBE ME AS:

_____

_____

_____

Common traits in outstanding leaders

We've worked with outstanding leaders across different sectors and have found that no matter the industry, there are always key qualities they have in common.

But let's focus on care leaders, as we were involved in some research in 2017 that looked specifically at care home managers from Outstanding rated homes. If you were a bit stuck on answering any of the questions in the last section, then this research should help you to consider your own qualities and benchmark yourself.

Achieving an Outstanding rating from CQC, we know is a team effort, but there had never been a lot of focus on the specific common qualities of the managers who had led their team to this coveted rating.

We teamed up with Article Consulting, who led the research to find out in more detail if there was anything that made these managers different, and if there was, then what could be learnt from them.

Here are some of the facts about the participants from the research:

- 81% of the managers were women.
- None of the managers had been in post for less than a year. Most had been in post for 1-5 years.
- 69% of the managers managed homes with 20-40 beds.
- Most of the participants managed a single, independent home or were part of a group with less than 10 homes.

Whilst the above are all factors you can have no real control of, here are some facts that you may have some control of:

- 78% of the managers had accessed networking events in the last 12 months.

- 72% had taken external training and the average was 6-10 days of formal training within the last 12 months.
- Most said that they had autonomy in how their home was run.
- Most said that they have regular reviews and share learnings with their staff.

The managers were asked what they believed had contributed the most to their Outstanding rating and 90% highlighted activity relating to staff, such as recruiting the right staff, providing adequate training and empowerment, and valuing staff members. They also attributed their Outstanding rating in part, to their effective and consistent leadership and creating a positive culture.

Regarding the top three qualities that the manager of an Outstanding rated care home needs to have, the qualities most frequently highlighted by respondents included: 'passionate' (71%), 'caring' (53%), 'dedicated' (41%) and 'a "can do" attitude' (41%).

You can read the full report on this research by heading to **www.careleadershandbook.co.uk**.

The difference in Outstanding managers

The second part of the research involved the managers taking the Judgement Index online assessment, which measures values-based behaviours, and that includes external behaviours (at work) and internal behaviours (in self) across over 60 areas.

The assessment is not a survey. It doesn't ask questions in a typical way that you may have experienced if you've taken assessments such as personality tests.

We will talk a bit more about the assessment much later in the book, but you don't need to have taken it yourself to consider what the assessment found and reflect on how you may compare to these managers.

This is what the results found:

Thinking strategically

The Outstanding managers had balance between their people skills, task processing skills and strategic thinking. This is actually pretty rare, as most people are in the here and now, thinking about **who** they are working with and **what** they are doing, rather than thinking strategically about their business. Lots of people think that they are strategic thinkers, especially CEO's and board members, but in fact, not many naturally are.

Imagine you are in a meeting and someone is talking about a project. Where do your thoughts first go? Most will begin by thinking about either **who** is involved in the project (the people aspects) or **what** the process, steps or tasks relating to the project are.

Although we should, we often fail to think outside the box about the wider implications. Perhaps this is down to our workload and other distractions, and therefore people often don't tap into that part of their brain. This finding with the Outstanding managers highlighted that being able to see the bigger picture in the working world, potentially has had a positive impact on their Outstanding result.

A tip:

The next time you're in a meeting, scribble the words "Big P" somewhere in the corner of your notepad and circle it. As the meeting progresses come back to those words and start thinking about the bigger picture of whatever is being discussed. What are the benefits? What are the consequences? Just remembering to tap into this way of thinking on a regular basis can help strengthen strategic thinking.

Problem solving

Three-quarters of the Outstanding managers scored as 'extremely capable' in their problem-solving ability and their capacity to understand, process and make decisions at pace. We think of this as the speed at which someone operates, and this suggests that these managers' ability to quickly think on their feet has been a key factor in their becoming Outstanding.

Problem solving is a skill that can be developed and it's fair to say that if you're in a job where you already have good knowledge and skills, your problem solving pace is bound to be quicker than if you didn't have good knowledge and skills.

An important thing to think about here, is what could slow down your problem solving pace? It tends to be stress and pressure. If you think about it, when you're stressed you tend to operate under a bit of a cloud of fog and that can make it harder to solve problems and make decisions. We may all get the odd day like that, but if stress or undue pressure is affecting you consistently then it's time to address it. We will talk more about stress shortly.

Other areas of strength

Some of the other strengths in the Outstanding managers, which were to be expected were:

- Strong intuition and capacity for noticing and sensing things.
- Strong precision and attention to detail.
- Healthy levels of self-criticism. They were not overly tough or negative on themselves.

The self-criticism finding is interesting because people often defend themselves if they are very self-critical, saying that it is important for maintaining their high standards.

Actually, we've often found that when people are overly self-critical it directly impacts on self-confidence and self-esteem, which is never good for someone's wellbeing.

A high level of self-criticism can also spill out into negativity onto others and drive a bad culture.

A tip:

If you find yourself consistently beating yourself up for not completing everything on your list or find that the words you use in your head to talk to yourself are negative, then it's time to take some action.

Give that self-critical voice in your head a name. Let's say Lesley. Whenever you're being too tough on yourself then tell that voice: "Thank you for your opinion Lesley, but these are all the great things I have completed today." Or "Thank you Lesley but I'm actually very good at my job because of these reasons."

By raising your awareness to when the voice is kicking in and addressing it, you'll find that Lesley appears less and less...

Energy for self vs energy for work

Probably the clearest, consistent finding from the assessment results was regarding the time and energy the Outstanding managers invested into themselves. The results showed that the managers were very good at putting energy back into themselves personally, which is rarely seen across a group like this. Why is it rare? Well, particularly in care we find that a person's energy will go to everyone else; their staff, the clients, their family and the last person on the list is themselves.

Think about how good you are at looking after you. What percentage of your energy goes to others versus the energy you put back into yourself? This can be taking time for yourself outside of work and doing something that fulfils you. It's not necessarily all about going to the gym or eating healthily, although that can play into it, but it's about what you give yourself versus others.

Across all industries, we find people are much better at giving their energy to others or to work, and not as good at directing energy to themselves. But 100% of the Outstanding managers were good at taking time and directing that energy to themselves. This is clearly an important finding.

Sometimes people find this concept a little difficult to understand, so we created a visual model to help bring it to life.

Imagine a two-tiered wedding cake. The top tier is labelled "work" and the bottom tier is labelled "self" and ideally the bottom tier would be wider and fatter or at least as wide as the top tier in order to provide a solid foundation to support the top one.

Most people's wedding cakes are actually reversed. The top tier will be the wider tier; the energy is all going to work or external factors and the self tier will be very skinny, neglected or unstable. Whilst this is common, and most people can go on for some time operating like this, there is always a danger of the wedding cake collapsing or toppling over if that bottom tier is not a strong foundation that can support the top one.

tHE WEDDING CAKE tHEORY

IDEAL WEDDING CAKE:

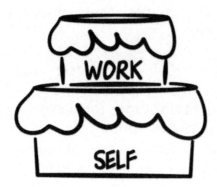

WHAT MOST PEOPLE'S WEDDING CAKE WOULD LOOK LIKE:

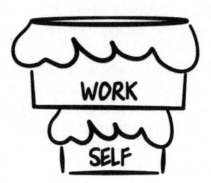

What would your wedding cake look like? We think that this is a really good thing to stay conscious of, and if you find you're having too many days, weeks or months where the self tier (your foundation) is being neglected then it's time to address what you can change to put more energy back in to you.

Our research and many other studies have found that people perform better at work when that foundation of self is solid. People like this are more likely to look after themselves, have good self-esteem, will not be too critical of themselves and will have a self-assured quality that allows them to bring their whole selves to work and perform to a high level.

The next time you realise you need to put more into **you** then don't feel guilty. Remember: You'll perform better at work as a result.

Strengths that can turn into barriers to performance

It's fair to say that 100% of the Outstanding rated managers had strong results from their assessments. But with strengths there can come potential 'spikes' or what we often call 'high performance frustrations' that can get in the way of someone performing at their best or getting the best from others.

A strength can be either positive or negative. It's like a superpower, it can be used for good or bad! We sometimes find that when someone is particularly strong in a certain area, for example let's say their precision to detail, then they will often expect the same meticulous precision from others, and that can cause great frustration if the team around them are not as precise or accurate as they are, especially if there could be genuine room for flexibility.

Some of the common barriers we find in care leaders are:

Resistance to ask for help

We see this across the care industry, not just with the Outstanding managers. If you're strong at solving problems for yourself and processing things in your head, you may find you resist asking for help. If you feel that you are a capable and independent problem solver, then you may feel you don't need help from others, or you may actively resist it, but it's worth considering if this strength ever turns into a "spike".

Do you resist asking for help when in fact, sometimes you could use some? If so, it's worth having a chat with your manager and the people who support you. If a manager knows to ask you: "Out of all the things you don't need help with, what's the one thing you **could** use some help with" and coerce it out of you, then that could make a great difference to your working life. We see this trait in so many care leaders, so take some time to think if this is you.

Tendency to take on too much

It's easy to fall into the trap of taking on too much, especially at work, and it's even more common in high performers like the Outstanding managers because they are constantly striving to do more and achieve more.

The danger of taking on too much and saying yes to everything or setting goals that are too big is that it can quite often lead to burnout, which we will come on to soon. This can often link with the resistance to ask for help, which we've just looked at and often you might be someone who thinks: "No one can help as I do it best." If this is the case, then it's time to sit down and evaluate as you might just be heading for burnout!

Precision to detail

As we've already mentioned, having a very meticulous nature and precision to detail can get in the way if you expect it from others when it's not necessary.

Granted in care there are many occasions when precision to detail is vital, particularly when dealing with medication or important paperwork, but consider whether your own precision is making you inflexible and may stop you from delegating work or whether the level of precision you like and have is unnecessary at times. Again, holding onto work because of meticulous standards could lead to burnout.

Potential to burn out

Most of the managers assessed for the research had a susceptibility to burnout, attributed to their high motivation levels and strong work ethic. This finding was supported by many of them highlighting in the survey that challenges faced in trying to achieve an Outstanding rating were managed through working extremely hard.

If you find yourself agreeing that you do tend to take on too much, struggle to ask for help and hold on to work in order to get it completed to the standards you want then you may well be susceptible to burnout.

How long do you think you can maintain these behaviours? At some point when you're spinning so many plates, those plates may start to fall. It's very similar to the wedding cake theory we used earlier. It's important to have the support in place to ensure that these strengths and 'spikes' you may have don't end up becoming barriers to performance.

We hope that highlighting these strengths has been useful for you to reflect on and consider your own. Remember – strengths are only positive if they are used in the right way.

Managing stress – a key skill for any leader

One of the most important findings in the Outstanding managers was their capacity to cope with stress, or let's say the resilience they had to deal with it both in their working world and in their personal world.

That's not to say that they did or didn't have stress. We know the job of a manager in any care organisation has enormous pressures. But the results showed that they were able to cope and maintain a positive attitude around any stress they may have had, and this can have a huge impact on someone's overall performance.

Think about your own behaviour when you're under a lot of stress or pressure. It may feel like a thick cloud of fog has come down over you and that can affect many different aspects of your work.

Typically, we find stress affects the following areas:

- Intuition – which can weaken.
- Problem solving – which may become slower.
- Strategic thinking – people who are under stress do not tend to tap into their strategic ability.

On the self-side, personal stress can impact on our self-confidence, our self-regard and sense of worth. When someone is under stress at both work and home then there really is no escape, and performance can obviously take a nosedive.

An important question to ask yourself if you are under stress or pressure and you recognise that it's affecting your performance, is what can you do to remove the stress from you or remove yourself from it? More of this soon when we look at resilience.

The science behind stress

At a conscious level our brain can typically process around seven pieces of information, give or take two bits, when it's working normally, thinking logically and we are not under any stress at all. But when stress is added and we become emotional our brain starts to lose the ability to process information. The more stress and uncontrollable negative emotion we have, the fewer bits of information we can process.

This is because our brain has gone into 'fight or flight' mode and is trying to protect us by only letting tiny bits of information get through. The problem with this is that by not taking in enough information, we can miss things and make mistakes.

Bear in mind that we may not be able to avoid a stressful scenario, but we could control our emotions whilst we deal with the stress. Being stressed and emotional is a dangerous combination and it goes without saying that most of the time, when we get stressed we also get emotional.

There will always be events and scenarios that can cause stress in our lives, but if we can handle them with resilience then we will be better equipped to cope with any periods of stress that may arise.

For now, reflect on how you handle stress and how it impacts on your emotions. We are going to share some strategies to handle stress and runaway emotions later in the book.

The power of resilience

"The capacity to absorb pressure and to recover quickly from difficulties; toughness and grit"

As we've discovered, the Outstanding rated managers seemed to have an ability to cope with any stress or pressure they were under, to a greater level than we normally see in care leaders. This means that they must have stronger levels of resilience, and this has been a key factor in their success and overall results.

Resilience is currently a buzz word and organisations are waking up to the fact that if people are not resilient, their wellbeing and subsequent performance will be at risk and this can impact on a whole range of organisation issues. Of course, the care sector is no different, but in care the other important consideration is vulnerable clients who are the heart of the service.

So, what is resilience?

Rob says: "You may relate the word to physical activities and coincidentally as I write this today, Sophie, my co-author and daughter has just finished a half marathon on very little preparation due to work and injury. You could say she showed both physical and mental resilience, especially as many in that situation wouldn't have made it to the start line."

Resilience has many forms and we can be resilient at different levels and in various ways. You may have the resilience to do a physical challenge, such as a Tough Mudder and have good mental determination and grit to complete it, but if you were asked to do something such as speak in public then this could see your resilience disappear as you hide in the nearest cupboard!

This would show that your confidence and emotional resilience were not as strong in that particular type of scenario. Regardless of the type of resilience, it can all be invested in and trained to become stronger.

One of the root issues within society today is that we are failing to develop resilience in our children. It became fashionable a few years ago to ban competition in schools for fear of upsetting children. The fact is, as you start to stretch children; providing it's in a safe and controlled environment they learn to cope and be more resilient.

The same is true regarding failure and god forbid we let little Johnny fail! However, we fail as a society and as parents if we don't teach children how to fail. It has built a culture of blame and lack of responsibility and over the past two decades may have contributed to a generation of people who just don't cope that well and are less resilient in many environments.

Regardless of age, background or generation we can develop resilience and coping mechanisms. We can also develop our care staff and leaders to help them get better at dealing with the various challenges that the care sector and indeed life throws at them.

The biggest areas of concern within the care and social sector tend not to be around physical resilience (although we are aware of how physically demanding the environment can be), but the emotional and stress related demands of the job.

Combined with stress at work, personal issues can affect anyone at any given time and our research has shown that over 30% of care staff working in under-performing care companies have moderate to high levels of personal stress. When compared with Outstanding rated care home managers the difference was significant as the Outstanding managers had very little work or personal stress in comparison. Remember we are not saying they had no stress, but that they had an ability to cope with any stress, whether that be at work or in their personal life.

Considering these differences in the groups it suggests that some care professionals have better coping mechanisms and resilience than others. It's clear that being able to be resilient both at work and at home can help us succeed, and so being able to identify our weaker resilience spots and put effort into developing them can make a difference.

To start, why not identify what areas you may be less resilient in. These could be:

- Personal home stress such as relationships, debt, children or family issues.
- Work stress such as working relationships, volume of work, technical and skill factors, confidence.
- Health and general fitness. For example, are there health or other medical issues that impact on your resilience?

The more areas that you are currently struggling in can have a bigger impact on overall resilience and performance.

Follow the steps below to take initial action:

Tips for building resilience

1. Identify your vulnerable areas to stress and pressure.
2. Avoid seeing any crisis as an insurmountable problem, you just need to find a pathway.
3. Rationally review and challenge the source of pressure or stress, identifying what you can influence and what you cannot. Note that it's rare to not be able to influence the source of the problem in some way.
4. Prioritise what is important and put your effort in that direction. Side-line things that are not critical and that drain your energy reserves.
5. Accept that change is a part of life and you may have to change.
6. Create a strategy and take action toward your goals. Use the GROW model which you will find later in the book.
7. Expose yourself to pressure in a controlled way so that you build coping mechanisms and stress control.
8. Nurture a positive view of yourself. Right now you are highly likely to be giving all your energy to others and work and neglecting yourself and this can leave you vulnerable.
9. Create a support network of people to help you build resilience. This does not mean abdicate responsibility; results come down to you.
10. Maintain a positive outlook and attitude and take control. To quote Nike: Just do it!

Building resilience is a key lesson in self-leadership and we hope that understanding more about the Outstanding rated managers and their own resilience has helped you to reflect and benchmark yourself. Whilst we've covered some simple steps above, there will be more exercises throughout the book which will help strengthen your resilience in different areas. The next step with this is to understand the relationship between mindset, emotions and behaviour.

If you've not taken a break yet whilst reading, now might be a good time to put the book down. Reflect on what you've noted and had your awareness raised to so far and let that sink in. We've seen how raising awareness alone can cause positive shifts in people, and perhaps you're already thinking about how you might start your day differently tomorrow.

When you're ready, we've got the last part of self-leadership to cover.

Mindset, emotions and behaviour

Rob says: *"Without doubt, when I was first introduced to the close relationship between mindset, emotions and behaviour during my studies and research it had a massive impact on me. In fact, it made me realise that when I had performed really well, the reason why that had likely happened and when things hadn't gone well, again, the reason why!*

This also translated across many aspects of my life including my career, personal life and sports life. Both good and bad performances nearly always came down to mindset and emotions and when I didn't get the results that I was capable of, it generally came down to me."

When we share these concepts as a module in our leadership academy it is always a memorable part of the course and this is because we put the delegates into what we call 'stretch' (not physical!). In order to truly understand how our mindset impacts on our emotions and then our behaviour we have to take our delegates out of their comfort zone. How do we do this? Well, we'd like to keep it a secret in case you ever end up on one of our workshops. But let's just say it involves a little bit of Elvis!

To put it into perspective without giving it away, think about something that would really take you out of your comfort zone. It could be doing a presentation in front of an audience. It could be having to deal with local authorities. It could be something in your personal life, like going on a first date or a lunch with your mother in law. Think about what your mindset is on any of these occasions, and how that might affect your emotions. How do your mindset and emotions then affect your behaviour? Let's explore all of this in more detail.

The clever thing about The Performance Spiral (which is the relationship between mindset, emotions and behaviour) is that it doesn't just reflect you in work, it can be used to reflect against all areas of your life. It can also be a social reflection and can be used with teams, your family and all aspects of human performance.

Care leaders find this module useful because it helps them measure and benchmark themselves, their teams and even the whole company. Once measured you can start to prioritise areas of intervention and in doing so create a powerful action plan to shape and develop yourself and your people. The spiral becomes a very practical performance tool and framework.

As you are guided through the model start to consciously rate yourself against the different areas and get a feel for how they impact on each other. Aim to have the spiral etched in your mind so that when you enter various scenarios you understand what is going on behind the action that's taking place. This will give you an ability to either maintain performance if it's good or intervene with an appropriate strategy; and we will share the strategies in the book as you work your way through it.

The Performance Spiral model

Let's start with the centre and end point of the spiral, which is the result or goal. Think about what sort of goals you currently have and what results you are getting. Are they good, bad or indifferent? Consider what aspects of life, work or even your organisation do these goals and results relate to? You could be getting great results in work but poor results in your personal life.

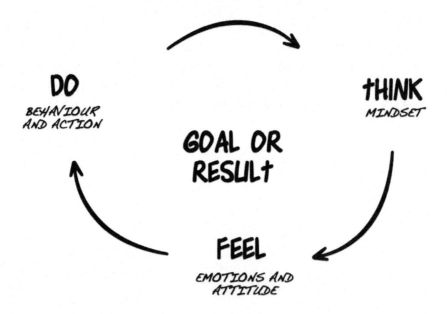

There is a whole section further on in the book looking at goals, goal setting and results in depth so to avoid repeating too much let's just run through a quick summary on goals to allow you to reflect.

Goals and results

Goals need to be quantified to a standard of what is good or bad and this gives an ability to measure the result. Far too often leaders fail to accurately communicate the quality or standard required in the goal and this can lead to them never being satisfied with the result.

It's also important to reflect **what** we do and **how** we react when we get the result and whether we take responsibility for it, which goes for both good and bad results.

The sad truth is that when we get a bad result we typically blame and deflect responsibility to someone or something: "It was the CQC's fault" or "The relatives of the client are so difficult." You may have said sentences to this effect on occasion? However, there is nearly always something we could have done from an action point which would have affected the result.

Another common phrase you may use with a bad result is: "In hindsight I would have done things differently" and this suggests you fail to take responsibility as a leader for spotting the potential issue ahead. In contrast, great leaders tend to have 'foresight' which helps them change course and put things in place to avoid failure and instead create a win or good result.

With good results, we tend to shy away from celebrating them and this echoes the comments we often hear from within the care sector. Many tell us that they do not get adequate praise for the great things they do, but know all too well, loud and clear about any mistakes and bad results. It may be a British, cultural thing to not make a fuss when we have done something fantastic. We find when we are working in the USA and our colleagues and clients over there get good results, we certainly know about it!

Take a moment to reflect on these questions:

- Are your goals quantified to a standard or quality?
- Do you or whoever relevant take responsibility for both success and failure?

• What strategy can you put in place to allow foresight and spot issues ahead?

Now let's move in reverse order around the spiral and review each step:

Do – Behaviour and action

Simply put, your actions and behaviour will be the deciding factor on your results. Therefore, have a think again about the sorts of results you are getting and consider what actions are being taken to get you those results.

When things go badly, the chances are that you didn't take quality action. Your behaviour was most-likely inconsistent. You may not have carried out actions in the correct order and sequence.

This is the point where you should take responsibility and reflect deeply about what you could do differently next time. Don't go back into the blame mindset, instead, be willing to change, because if you don't you will continue to get bad results.

When things go well and there is a good result you'll find you probably followed an order and sequence, behaved consistently in order to achieve the goal and took quality action which determined the good result.

A good way of relating this, is to think about weight loss. You could have the correct mindset and attitude about losing weight, but ultimately, if you do not take quality and consistent action, if you're not consistent in your healthy eating and exercise and don't follow some kind of plan, then the result won't be good. This is a great opportunity to have a think about what you could do to increase the quality and consistency of your actions in certain scenarios.

Feel – Emotions and attitude

Let's start with some simple definitions because in our training we often ask people to define what they think an attitude is and they normally just focus on a bad attitude.

Attitude – A pre-disposition to think, feel and act in a certain way to a scenario. In short, we have learned and shaped our attitudes. We are not born with set attitudes, but through life we may develop attitudes that drive our behaviour, either positively or negatively. This also has an impact directly on emotions.

To be clear, people are not born with pre-dispositioned attitudes. They are not automatically homophobic, racist, or dislike the colour purple. These attitudes are shaped through experience or other influences and can change over time.

Emotion – Emotions run deeper than attitudes and are triggered by your senses. Once triggered your attitude kicks in and based on your emotion or feelings towards the scenario your attitude will be directed either positively or negatively.

Emotions are inbuilt and research tells us that we have around twenty-seven possible emotions, ranging from anger or disgust to admiration and joy. There are also a variety of responses that go with these emotions.

One of the first things we talk about during our leadership academy is that if you want movement in your people then you need to create emotion. The clue is in the word itself: 'E - Motion'. Yes, the word is motion which suggests movement. The more movement required, then the more emotion you need to generate in those you wish to move. Here lies the link to motivation which you will learn more about later in the book.

As mentioned, because attitudes are learned and shaped, they can be re-shaped if needed. Emotions are fairly well housed within us but can definitely be impacted on and either contained if needed, or released to create behaviour and movement.

Now here is the potential issue: What happens when you have a negative attitude to a certain scenario or someone you work with? We hear the same complaints from leaders in all different industries about the negative attitudes and emotions of their staff and it's funny how we hear the same complaints from workers about their bosses!

How much wasted time do you spend on people in your team with negative attitudes or poorly controlled emotions? Imagine what you could do with the spare hours, but also imagine the impact on morale within your organisation if all the negative attitudes and emotions were removed.

Now, this is where it starts to liven up, so again we ask you to reflect for a moment on the bad results you may be getting. Link the result to the actions and behaviour that may not be up to the quality they should be, and now consider how emotions and attitude may have impacted negatively on those actions.

Likewise, do this for the great results you are getting and think what your mood was like before taking action to get the good result. Were you motivated, excited, in control and with a positive attitude? We can bet on it. When you have a good attitude and positive emotions, you're much more likely to take the positive actions in order to get the good result.

We find the biggest negative influences on attitude and emotions are external factors, such as someone else's opinion or judgement.

So, ask yourself this: **Who owns your attitude and emotions?**

Yes, you! But how often do you let something, or someone else take hold of them and influence them? Who in your company for example, do you not get on with, and how much does that feeling and attitude you have about them impact on your performance? The reason why we reference who you may not get on with is because many will blame someone else when things don't go well: "It was their fault, as they put me in a bad mood and I didn't perform well."

Think about the word **mood**.

Mood is a description of an emotion and who owns it? You!

You should be getting the concept of the spiral now and starting to understand the impact of emotions and attitudes on performance. For now, let's continue with the spiral.

Think - Mindset

The influence our state of mind has on how we think and feel emotionally has been researched and well documented. We all will have been in scenarios where we've had either a positive or a negative mindset. Looking at the spiral we can see that our mindset will influence the outcome or result, so let's consider the key elements of mindset and the influence it has on our attitude and emotions and in turn, our actions.

Vision

Firstly, our vision of the outcome of a scenario will have a dramatic impact on our emotions and attitude.

Let's say your regional manager is on their way to visit your home and you don't get on that well. If you did get on then you may form a vision of a successful day, however in this scenario and if you don't get on then you may see a bad day ahead which will affect your emotions negatively and drive a bad attitude about the day. Another example could be something like a snap inspection or an outbreak of illness. What would you visualise in one of those scenarios? Whatever it is, whether your vision is of success or failure, it will influence emotions and attitude either positively or negatively.

Belief

Prior to this, embedded in your long-term memory may be beliefs that have been formed through knowledge and experience. Beliefs can either be positive, empowering beliefs that then influence a positive vision, or negative, limiting beliefs that create a vision of failure.

You might wonder why anyone would have a limiting belief, but they are inbuilt within us and designed to protect us from doing things such as stepping out into oncoming traffic or trying to stroke a lion. The limiting belief signals danger and stops us from doing things that could cause us harm. The problem is that limiting beliefs can go into overdrive, dominate and be formed from poor evidence.

You may have been told by someone once that you wouldn't be good at doing a task or that something bad was going to happen and perhaps you believed them, but their opinion could have been incorrect or based on inaccurate facts. Yet if that opinion influenced you to not try something then it influenced your mindset, emotion and behaviour and this is how powerful your beliefs can be in your spiral.

Self-Image

Another element within the spiral that sits firmly within your mindset is your self-image. Your self-image is simply a reflection of how you see of yourself, and this can change depending on the scenario or event you are in.

Think about times when you know you are good at something you are about to do - Perhaps comforting a particular client who is upset. Your self-image would probably be high at this point, because you know you can handle the scenario and do a good job.

On the flip side, think of a situation such as having to give a speech in public or sing karaoke at the Christmas party! Yes, there will be a few who can't wait to break into a bit of Elvis or Chaka Khan, but for many the thought of this will create a very low self-image in their minds.

Poor self-image can drive a limiting belief, which can drive a vision of failure. This overall mindset then drives a poor attitude and negative emotions which then contribute to poor action and behaviour, resulting in a bad result. Ok, this is a bit of a mouthful, but this now gives the full picture of the complete spiral.

Take a look at the full spiral now and all of the elements that sit within it. Every single one of these has the ability to spin the spiral up or down.

Looking at it like this we appreciate that the spiral looks quite complicated, so in the next section we've broken it down into a real-life scenario to demonstrate how the spiral can either go up or down, depending on the elements within it.

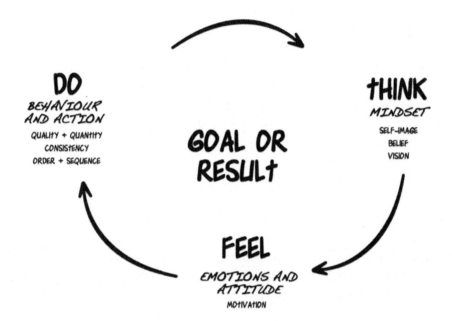

THE PERFOMANCE SPIRAL

DO
BEHAVIOUR AND ACTION
QUALITY + QUANTITY
CONSISTENCY
ORDER + SEQUENCE

GOAL OR RESULT

THINK
MINDSET
SELF-IMAGE
BELIEF
VISION

FEEL
EMOTIONS AND ATTITUDE
MOTIVATION

The Spiral in action

At this point it's worth saying that in a real-life scenario the spiral can happen very quickly, and our mindset, emotions and behaviour can almost become a blur rather than a sequence. To some extent our emotions are picking up on things through our senses before we have even registered them in our minds.

However, for simplicity and to illustrate the model let's take the sequence in order and we are going to use an example of a scenario you could have been in or may find yourself in at some point in the future.

The scenario

Your home has won an award for outstanding care and contribution to the community and you must give an interview to the local press for the evening news, but you are totally unprepared and get really nervous whenever you have to speak in public or have the spotlight on you.

What could potentially happen to your spiral?

Downward spiral

Self-image - is low because you do not think you are good at public speaking and have spent the whole day running around so feel a bit frazzled and dishevelled.

Belief - is limiting because you were once told by a teacher that you would never be a good public speaker.

Vision – is of failure and you imagine yourself stumbling over your words and people saying mean things about you.

Emotions and attitude – your attitude is negative and you become emotional.

Motivation – you cannot motivate yourself to prepare properly because emotions have taken over.

Action – because you are feeling emotional your actions are of poor quality and you stumble over your words in the interview and forget key points.

Result – a poor result! And then you communicate and reinforce the negative message to yourself by saying: "I'm rubbish at public speaking and I never believed I would do a good job."

Now let's consider if this spiral was reversed:

Upward spiral

Self-image – is high because you have done similar things before and know you deserve to be doing this interview.

Belief - is empowering as you have done this before and are comfortable speaking and controlling yourself while you speak. People have also told you that you've done a great job in the past, which reinforces your empowering belief.

Vision – you can see the great headlines about your company clearly in your mind and the feeling of pride coming from your team.

Emotions and Attitudes – your attitude is that of being 'up for it' and you have positive, happy emotions.

Motivation – you are highly motivated and start to take action by rehearsing your speech and key interview points.

Action – you produce a quality interview and speech. You take time to celebrate your achievement. You say to yourself: "I knew I would nail it, I saw it and believed I would get a good result!"

THE OUTCOME

These two entirely different outcomes become self-fulfilling prophecies. Did you recognise the patterns in any situations you've found yourself in recently? Have you seen this happen to people around you, in your team?

In a care environment you may find that the spiral kicks in many times in a day, not just in bigger scenarios like the example we've described. As well as individual spirals there can also be the collective spiral of the entire team. Consider that the momentum of the spiral and whether it spins upwards or downwards is always within your power.

The next time you're at work, try and look at scenarios unfolding and spot what's happening to the spiral. If it's a downward spiral and you can identify the point in the spiral that's the problem, then you have a chance at getting stuck in with an intervention and reversing the spiral.

For example, you may see that belief is the issue which has started a downward spiral in someone on your team. Or perhaps it's the vision of the entire team if you're working towards something like a CQC inspection. If you can pinpoint exactly what on the spiral is causing it to spin downwards, then you have a chance to do something about it and change its direction.

Within the book we will focus on interventions and mechanisms to create positive, powerful, upward spirals in life and work with the aim that you can improve confidence, emotional control, commitment and communication, for both yourself and your people. Keep the spiral in the back of your mind and refer to it again and again as you need to.

Leading Yourself – Summary

Now that you've had a good reflection of yourself and understand what can impact on your performance it's time to move into the next part of the book; leading others. This next chunky section will have more practical exercises to go and work on with your team, but don't forget to come back to yourself and make that investment when you need to.

Keeping your awareness raised as to where you are on the spiral, your resilience levels, and what your development or potential strengths that can be "spikes" are will help to support you as a good leader moving forward.

This first section should have set you up for the rest of the book and in the future you will meet many people and leaders that will not have this level of understanding that you now have.

Remember it's you who has the ownership and power to continue to grow and develop if you want to.

Part 2

Leading Others

Emotional intelligence

Have you heard of emotional intelligence or EQ before? It's one of the most significant human qualities needed within the care sector and anyone who is a fantastic manager or care professional is likely to have high levels of emotional intelligence. Like any intelligence it can be developed, so let's explore **what** it is, **why** it's so important and **how** to develop it in yourself and your people.

When people think about intelligence it often conjures up thoughts of someone being smart, articulate, perhaps good at puzzles and maths problem-solving. However, there are many different types of intelligences, at least sixteen have been defined.

An example of a type of intelligence is people who are very self-aware of their body positioning and controlling movement when flying through the air. A gymnast has very good 'bodily kinaesthetic intelligence'. In contrast you may find someone who is clumsy and falls over a lot may not have very good spacial awareness and therefore will not have very good kinaesthetic intelligence.

Another example would be people who have a very naturalistic type of intelligence like horse whisperers and people who connect very well with animals.

> ***Rob says:*** *"When I was a kid, I had a friend called Carl and when he came to our house our friendly pet Labrador, Ash, would simply want to attack him. Was Carl just not naturally gifted when it came to animals? Or did Ash know something we didn't know?!"*

Putting this back into the care environment, just take a few moments to think about which members of your team really connect and naturally engage with people and who might not be so natural.

Have another think about which members of staff are highly emotional and don't necessarily control their own emotions well as this plays into emotional intelligence which we will share more about shortly.

What about you? What are your intelligence strengths? How well do you control your emotions day to day?

Emotional intelligence definition

So, let's define what EQ is and where it has evolved from. Emotional intelligence has always existed, but has only in recent decades been defined and its significance understood. In the 90's a science journalist called Daniel Goleman realised that being successful wasn't down to being typically IQ-type clever. His book 'Emotional Intelligence' was on the New York Times Best Seller list for over 18 months, as people were so eager to understand more about how they could develop their own EQ and get ahead in the workplace.

Think about it, you may know someone who could spell compassion but lacks it! In short, IQ is not enough alone to define success. Having worked in the care sector for a number of years, we've seen that it's critical to have good EQ ability and it's never a surprise when we analyse high performers at any level within care, that they tend to have a high degree of EQ even if they didn't know it at the time.

So, what is it? To start, we need to go back and look deeper into emotions and what they are. There are reported to be twenty-seven different types of emotion and they have been formed within us through evolution for the purpose of moving us either toward something, or away from something. That's why we see the word 'motion' within emotion, as we covered earlier in the book.

In this way, emotions are critical for our movement and to spur us on to take action. A problem can occur when we are not in control of our emotions and they take over our mind and body, often creating mayhem internally or for others around us.

Can you think of any incident when you've 'lost it' emotionally and behaved inappropriately? How did your emotions create mayhem for you internally and result in you taking a bad action on something?

If this is something you personally feel you need to focus on, and your emotions have a habit of running away with you, then there is a fantastic book we recommend called "The Chimp Paradox" by Professor Steve Peters. The book uses the simple analogy of a 'chimp' to help you take control of your emotions and act in your own, best interest, whether it's in making decisions, communicating with others, or your health and happiness.

Emotional intelligence in detail

There are a number of more detailed definitions and models that explain EQ and you won't go far wrong by reading any of Daniel Goleman's work on EQ and leadership but let's start you off with two key areas; EQ within yourself, and EQ in a social context. Each of these areas has two sub-areas, a level of awareness and a level of management.

EQ

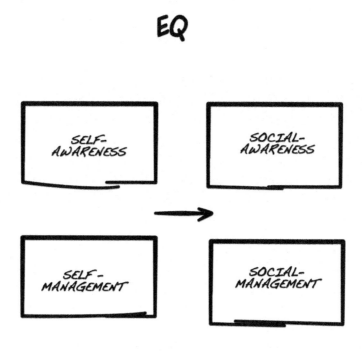

Self-awareness or personal EQ

Self EQ, or Self-awareness is when you have an understanding and awareness of where your emotions are at a given time. Let's imagine this as being aware of our inbuilt 'emotional Richter scale'.

For instance, imagine you are in a queue for the bathroom and someone pushes in front of you. You feel the blood rise up in your chest, your face goes red and you shout to the person that there is a queue and gesticulate wildly at the people patiently waiting. Suddenly, everyone is looking at you and you feel embarrassed for reacting in such a dramatic way.

Whether it was right or wrong for the person to push in, the question is: At what point did you become self-aware of your behaviour? If you had these reactions and only became aware when people started looking at you then it suggests you may not have as much self-awareness as someone who would be able to catch themselves before their reaction took over and deal with the situation in a more controlled way.

The importance of this is because if we are not aware of where our emotions are on the 'emotional Richter scale' then we are less likely to be able to control them. The word 'Richter' hopefully gives a good description of what out-of-control behaviour is like, if you think the of the tremors and earthquakes that some people produce when they lose it! You may have seen this in people who have a very short fuse and tend to boil over like a kettle on a stove. According to Professor Steve Peters, this is when 'the chimp takes over' and people like this will report after the incident of inappropriate behaviour, that they were unaware that they were starting to lose emotional control.

Self-management

Self-Management is about taking self-awareness to the next level and having the ability to regulate your emotions, mindset, stress or excitement and bodily responses to a point where you know you will perform best, in whatever context that is.

In our previous example, this could be taking a breath and handling the bathroom queue jumper in a firm but controlled manner; keeping your emotions in check and avoiding the dramatic outburst and red face.

In the care environment you may have to manage your emotions multiple times a day. It could be when comforting a resident, or taking an important exam, or handling conflict between two staff members. Depending on the scenario, you may need a high level of a certain emotion and other times you may need a much-reduced level, or to control a different emotion.

Have a think about how you perform best in certain scenarios and which emotions work best. How does your emotional Richter scale correspond with a great result that you have had? Perhaps you've performed well in a practical exam because you managed to control your nerves and emotions and stay calm when under pressure. No matter what the situation may be, the point is that being able to control and if necessary 'shift' or move your emotions, then your mindset and subsequent actions will reflect your level of EQ.

In summary, the 'self' part of EQ relates to you understanding what would lift and lower your emotions, being aware of where they are at any given point, understanding the ideal level and type of emotion required to perform at your best and then having the tools and ability to shift your own emotions to the desired state. Why not rate yourself in these various parts and ask your staff and friends how they would rate you. Be careful if you have this conversation with a partner though as it can be sensitive!

Social awareness or EQ

Now this is where the subject of EQ gets really interesting, especially for a leader as it includes not just you or a single person, but a group of people. Social EQ refers to how a group interacts to create emotions at the appropriate level to perform at the groups best within a given scenario.

An example might be at a team meeting, having a discussion, dealing with an incident or even just chilling out at a social event. The framework is the same as the 'self EQ' as it contains a level of awareness first and then the management of those emotions.

Social Awareness is the starting point and it comes down to an ability to read emotions from the way someone is communicating at a given time with either their body, energy or sound.

How good are you at reading someone in a situation and guessing where they are on their own emotional Richter scale? Are they pumped up and overly excited or maybe withdrawn and lacking the right emotion? This is the first level of social EQ and it's closely linked with empathy.

Add another layer to this and let's say that the person you are reading knows that you know where they are on the emotional Richter scale.

Now let's go even further and let's say the person also knows where you are on the emotional Richter scale and that you know that they know! Now you have total understanding and empathy between the pair of you.

Wow, we are getting complex here but have a think about the people you are really close to, the ones who you totally get and they get you. That is what we call a high level of Social EQ at an awareness level.

Now, think about how many people in your team and times it by itself. If you have six team members would be 6 x 6 = 36. This reflects the points of contact available within your team of six. That's a lot of mutual understanding that can potentially be developed and the chances are, right now you may only have that level of social awareness with one or two people in your team, if at all. Social awareness will have a direct reflection on team cohesion and performance, so the more of it you have, then better the team cohesion is likely to be.

Social management

Social management is the ability within a group of people to manage each other's emotions and a team who are good at this will have an ability to communicate and shift each other's emotions to an appropriate level for whatever function or scenario they need to perform in.

The key with this is understanding each other's emotional drivers, having an ability to communicate appropriately and knowing where each other needs to be on their respective emotional Richter scales.

If this is all available, then we are in a good place to influence each other to perform best. Therefore, to have the best chance of creating the right emotion we need to be both socially aware, with good EQ levels and then have the tools, communication and ability to shift people.

Take a moment to think about your team and reflect on how they perform together and what group emotions cause either an individual or the group to perform well or poorly. For instance, there could be a taboo subject or topic of conversation – perhaps politics, that you know will create undesirable emotions if certain people are in the room and subsequently the group emotions are driven down and the team don't communicate or perform well for the remainder of the day.

Sophie says: "Haven't we all teased someone to wind them up, knowing it will 'kick off'? I used to do this to my little sister when we were young. She had a fiery temper and I knew that if I said certain things to her or even looked at her the wrong way, that she would fly into a rage. It amused me a great deal at the time, but it is an example of how you can impact on the emotions of others if you know what buttons to push. This power can be used for good or bad!"

Flipping this concept, know that you have it in your power to influence and push buttons for good and create a great environment to perform. We always ask the groups we are training: "Who owns your attitude and emotions?" and they always state that they do, but remember it's not difficult for someone else to take control and create an environment of panic and anxiety which will inevitably result in a poor performance.

Again, thinking about the points of contact in a team of six (36), then this can be a challenging and complex area to improve, especially as emotions are infectious and if one person is in a bad or disruptive emotive state then it can impact on everyone.

To demonstrate how contagious this is, start your next team meeting by asking everyone to look at each other and pull a great big cheesy grin. Within seconds everyone will be grinning naturally and probably laughing for real! A live demonstration that emotions are infectious!

Controlling emotions and having great levels of EQ is essential to the cohesion and performance of your people and this will have a direct impact on many people factors such as the quality of care, attendance, discipline, wellbeing, professionalism and ultimately what your residents and clients think of you. And we all know that satisfaction and referrals from those you look after can mean a successful care organisation.

How to develop personal and social EQ

As we've mentioned, there are many books written on EQ and how to develop it. EQ is an important element in your leadership journey and this chapter may inspire you dive further into this subject. We wanted to summarise our top tips for awareness and management for both personal and social EQ, but bear in mind we are only scratching the surface here.

Self-awareness and management

Acceptance and responsibility

This is sometimes difficult, because when we behave inappropriately, we tend to blame something or someone else. You need to accept that you own your emotions so soak it up and take responsibility. The first step is ownership! Realise that outside influences do not and should not determine your emotions and behaviour. You have a choice to view things from a different perspective, and then consciously choose how you will respond.

Develop self-awareness

We are constantly monitoring our phones, appearance and other external factors. Yet, few of us monitor our thoughts, emotions, and behaviour to the same depth. Ask yourself throughout the course of your day how you are feeling.

Is the way that you are feeling negatively affecting your choices? Are you choosing your behaviours in an intelligent manner or allowing others to control and impact your emotional buttons? Start by reviewing your emotions at the start of the day and over the space of a few weeks gradually increase it to a number of set times. This will create a habit and you will soon be reviewing yourself and raising that level of awareness in a natural and consistent way.

Short fuses and impulses

Impulsiveness is a common cause of personal turmoil and can be caused by a lack of awareness as to where we are on the emotion Richter scale. We need to make an effort to steady the Richter scale before it's too late and we have done something impulsive like shouted at someone, had a glass of wine too many or whatever the impulse is that could lead to a bad result. This type of behaviour moves us further away from our objectives.

Notice when you are behaving in a counterproductive manner because you will no longer make effective choices. Stop sabotaging yourself. As soon as you are aware of unstable emotions then stop. Think: "What outcome do I really want in order to get a great result?" What emotion would you need to have to make that happen?

Physical

Whenever you feel your emotional Richter scale becoming unstable, a great physical practice is to immediately focus on your breathing technique. Take deep controlled breaths of around five seconds and on the out breath imagine blowing away the negative thought. On the next in-breath visualise what the emotion you'd like to have in a word, such as 'calm' and breathe that new emotion in!

Visualisation

Visualisation can be a very powerful tool. Having a bank of visual triggers; words and memories from when you have had a certain emotion in the past can be tapped in to, in order to release the emotion within you. Emotions carve a deep path to our memory, so if we trigger the memory, we also release the emotion, or at least a level of it.

Try this now: Consider when you have been super chilled and relaxed in the past and drill it down to the exact memory. It might be a holiday you had.

Where was it? What did it look like? Were there any smells, temperature and other senses that you can remember? Now, if you repeat the word 'relax' and play back the memory, a bit like a video in your mind, along with the senses you will effectively be able to release the emotion connected to the memory.

It takes practice and perseverance and visualisation is a technique used by the likes of sportsmen competing or medical surgeons about to operate. Once you have mastered this you should be able to say the word with a few breaths, quickly visualise yourself being emotionally relaxed and at the point on the emotional Richter scale that will get you a good result. This activity can be repeated with other memories connected to different emotions so that you have a bank of them to call on as scenarios present and require you to shift emotionally.

Social awareness and management

In order to have good social awareness and social management you need to have good self-awareness and self-management. Once you've got the self-side progressing positively then you're ready to look at other people and as a leader be able to step in and manage the emotions of someone who may not be aware of EQ and their emotional Richter scale.

Remember – emotions impact on behaviour. If you can manage, influence or control someone's emotions then you can influence outcomes in your people.

Active listening

Social awareness starts with being able to read and interpret the emotional state of someone and we can do this through 'active listening', a phrase often used by coaches and refers to listening with your whole body including ears, eyes and senses. Are you listening enough and if so, what are you picking up?

Rob says: "*Nothing frustrates me more than trying to communicate with people who do not listen and are constantly in 'send' mode rather than 'receive' and anyone who is ex-military may have heard of that phrase. This is an example of how a thought can manipulate emotions, as I can feel myself getting annoyed just thinking about this! Pause, breath, trigger word: 'relax', vision. I'm back!*"

A good way to listen is with your eyes by reading body language. People working in care tend to be good at this if they've worked with clients who can't communicate verbally but be cautious about coming to concrete conclusions regarding someone's body language unless you are experienced and understand what's normal for that person. Often assumptions can be made about body language, but just because someone scratches their nose it does not necessarily mean they are lying!

A good start to increase your active listening ability is simply to observe more. Start to watch colleagues more closely and look for shifts in body language, gestures, skin colour and breathing patterns that correlate with the emotion and behaviour you see. Over time this will help you to be aware and manage the emotions of colleagues, clients, friends and even children.

When someone is feeling pressured you might also see exaggerated personality traits being exhibited. Reserved or introvert types typically get more introverted and reserved when under pressure and in contrast the extrovert may become louder and try to dominate a situation. We will come back to personality types later as it's an interesting challenge to lead and manage different personality types.

Respond rather than react

When practicing building your social management skills keep the focus on responding. Those with lower levels of emotional intelligence tend to react, rather than respond. Responding requires thought and consideration. When you respond, you are making a conscious decision. Reacting is more of a knee-jerk reflex. There is little or no thought involved, just an emotional response.

EQ group exercise

To take this to another level with your team in a relaxed environment and run an observation session with them. Explain that you want individuals to share how they feel in certain scenarios and what their subsequent action and behaviour is. Have others reflect on what they observe about each other in these scenarios.

Use some typical examples such as a difficult family member or the local authority visiting, but also happy scenarios like a client's birthday or a staff party. Having people share how they feel in these scenarios and others sharing what they observe can start to create high levels of social awareness at a base level because if we are aware, we have an ability to act and change the dynamic of a scenario for the outcome we really want.

Leading on from developing a groups inter-personal observation you can also have individuals share how their colleagues might interact with them better to help shift their emotional Richter scale to the appropriate level with the right emotion.

Even with the best intentions we sometimes say or do the wrong thing that can send someone in the opposite emotional direction of what was intended. How many times have you told someone to calm down and they had the opposite reaction? We all respond differently, so, get to know each other and find out what works best.

Work at increasing your empathy. Those with high levels of emotional intelligence are skilled at recognising and relating to the emotions of others. Recognising that someone is upset will allow you to have a more effective and appropriate response. Ask yourself how you would like to be treated if you were feeling the same emotions.

You probably know someone highly skilled at managing their emotions. Their emphasis will always be on finding solutions. They refrain from getting angry or defensive. These individuals make intelligent decisions and can view themselves objectively. EQ is an important component of healthy relationships, both at home and at work. Your life will be more successful if you can effectively learn how to manage the emotions of yourself and others.

In order to have a team that functions with fantastic EQ then remember the example equation we shared earlier of a team of 6 having 36 points of contact. If everyone can be aware of and manage their own emotions and also be aware of and manage each other's emotions then you will have a team who can empathise and perform to a much higher level and many of the 'people problems' you experience and have to deal with as a leader will be gone.

State management – physical and emotional control

In our leadership academies we train students in techniques to manage emotions and behaviour so that they can perform to an optimal level and this is what we call 'state management'. Some people might refer to this as 'mental training' which it is in a way, but because it also includes physical action and the aim is to have mind, body and spirit acting in synchronicity we refer to it as 'state', rather than just mental.

When you become proficient at managing your state it can help you do many positive things. What it cannot do, however, is grant you skills if you do not possess them. You could be in the right state to sing like Andrea Bocelli but if you do not have the skills and technique to sing opera then don't expect good state management to be enough!

State management training is not a substitute for technical training, its primary purpose is to enable you to achieve your potential in any given scenario through the control of your emotions.

Think about when you've been in a scenario where you had the right level of emotions and behaviour to do a great job. Perhaps it was in a difficult meeting with the local authority? If you were in a situation that would normally make you nervous, or you'd get upset or frustrated but you handled the meeting really well, then the chances are you were in the right state to get a good result.

The science

The brain is divided into the conscious and the sub-conscious state. The sub-conscious is an incredibly powerful and complicated machine that mankind has barely begun to realise. It fulfils an amazing amount of functions, both physical (as a survival machine) and mental or emotional, with built in balances and checks.

We have already looked at emotional intelligence (or EQ) at length and you now understand the basics of awareness and management of emotions.

Your brain acts unconsciously to allow you to do many complex automated actions and reactions in a day, but it also reacts to messages from your conscious mind and sometimes your conscious mind can get it wrong. This is because the conscious mind is a state when you are aware of your thoughts, feelings and emotions and therefore they can influence your judgements and behaviour. In other words your conscious mind can be responsible for sending you into a downwards spiral as discussed earlier.

Let's give an example.
Do you ever leave your house and within a few minutes think: "Did I lock the door?" You then build the thought and belief and start to feel nervous about your house being unsecure. The next thing you know, you are running home in a panic only to find you had actually locked the door!

Regardless of how complex the brain and our mind is, it can be trained with very simple methods. The Chimp Paradox book, which we've already mentioned is dedicated to understanding this subject and uses the analogy of a chimp which acts as the emotional part of the brain. Everyone has a chimp but the extent of how it influences our actions can be varied depending on the control we have over it.

State management basics

In this section we have focused on just a few simple techniques that will help you control your state and allow you to perform at your best and control your emotions in order to deliver a fantastic result.

Five of the main aspects of state management are:

- Relaxation
- Visualisation
- Mental rehearsal
- Focus
- Positive affirmation

Relaxation

Progressive muscular relaxation (PMR) is one of sports most widely used techniques but can be used in any scenario and by anyone. If you know you have a situation coming up that could cause your emotions or behavior to get out of control and you have enough time beforehand then PMR should be used as a preliminary to both mental rehearsal and focusing on the situation ahead.

An example could be preparing yourself to give a verbal warning to a member of staff for something they've done wrong, that you are particularly angry or frustrated about. You may have had to do this or something similar where you will have wanted to keep your emotions in check.

The technique: You sit or lie in a relaxed position, start with some deep breathing and then systematically and progressively tense and relax your entire body from the feet upwards. This technique is without doubt the most effective ever created to relieve tension and allow you to focus and think logically. If you have time to do it before a meeting that you know will be stressful then it can make all the difference. It also helps if you're struggling to sleep!

Speed Relaxation

This technique is again widely used in sport but has also been successful with the military and uniformed services as people may have to manage their emotional and physical state from a heightened state such as running around carrying equipment, to a very calm and controlled state to perform a task.

You may have experienced something like this in care when there has been an emergency and people have to dash to a client, but then need a cool and measured mind and functioning physical state to deal with the emergency.

This technique can be used to slow down your heart rate or to relieve tension. With speed relaxation you concentrate solely on your arms and your legs using a technique called 'fives'. Why not try it now.

Fives Exercise

Firstly, assess your state, assess how calm and relaxed you are and what your heart rate is like.

Now: Whilst still seated on your chair take a couple of **deep** chest breaths to build up your oxygen level.

Then take another deep chest breath counting up from one to five in your mind:

1-2-3-4-5

Whilst you are counting you must **progressively** tense both your arms and your legs until they are at maximum tension by the count of five.

Now hold it... and hold it a little longer... then slowly breath out, counting down from five to one:

5-4-3-2-1

Progressively relaxing your tensed muscles as you exhale.

Now repeat the process once more and then re-assess your state and heart rate which will have hopefully dropped to a more relaxed and calm level. In a real-life scenario you may do this just once and very quickly before taking action. It's a moment of breath to gather yourself and your emotions before doing what you need to do.

Visualisation

What you see is what you get. We've already looked at visualisation in the Performance Spiral and it can also be referred to as visual rehearsal, self actualisation or imagery.

Since our evolution we have had the ability to produce visual images and pictures in our minds. The expression: "picture that in your mind's eye" is especially appropriate and is a very powerful means of supporting good performance, especially when a successful outcome is the vision.

Again, sport is a great example and many athletes will visualise a result prior to taking action, such as taking a penalty in football or hitting a golf shot. Search for a YouTube video of David Beckham before he is about to take a free kick (we recommend the clip of Greece 2001) and you will see him taking a moment to visualise the ball going into the back of the net.

The same works for care and if you are having to do something complicated or under pressure then visualising the process successfully first can help you to get a good outcome.

The reason this works is because the sub-conscious brain finds it very difficult to discern between something which has been imagined and something that has actually happened. All the brain knows is what has been programmed into it and by visualising something you want to happen you have programmed your sub-conscious into thinking it has done it already and therefore can repeat it when needed. Clever!

The technique behind visualisation is simply to relax and visualise yourself doing the task perfectly. Visualise it **through** your eyes as if you are **doing** the skill rather than watching yourself on a tv screen. When practising, visualise it in full colour HD and try to make that picture as clear as possible. Add any other senses you can think of including sound and smell to create a powerful 'real' scenario.

We know it sounds strange but it really works. Research has shown that athletes who have been injured and cannot compete but have trained visually during rehab lose very little skill, if at all in their performance when they start competing again.

Mental rehearsal

Mental rehearsal can condition your sub-conscious mind into expecting and anticipating what is going to happen and prepare it for the task to come. If, for example, you have to give a public speech to a group of strangers, your brain will get straight into gear because it thinks it has done it dozens of times before. The objective is for your sub-conscious mind to think: "Ah yes I recognise this situation, there is nothing to worry about, I know how to handle this."

Mentally picture yourself:

- On the morning of the public speech preparing yourself.
- Then waiting to be called forward for the speech.
- Going through the process.

And so on. Mentally prepare yourself for any eventuality, this is known as '**What if?**' scenario setting. Plan in advance what you are going to do if it rains, if the microphone doesn't work and how you will handle the questions from your audience. This is not being negative; it is foreseeing possible problems and working out a solution in advance, which can only be to your benefit.

Focus

Focusing should become part of your preparation routine if you know you have a situation, event or task coming up that you need to perform well and 'be on it'. The technique should be used prior to the event and whilst you are doing your mental rehearsal.

Choose a 'trigger' phrase or mantra at the start of the process to instantly remind you of the emotional state you need to be in for it. This could vary depending on the task, but we find our students often choose words such as 'energy', 'focus' or 'calm'.

The purpose of this technique is to send positive, well-established signals to your sub-conscious. You are programming it to give you the desired effect. The more you practice with your trigger word during your preparation sessions, the better you will be able to focus your attention during the actual event you are doing, simply by saying the trigger word in your head.

Positive affirmation

One of the biggest factors that undermines confidence is self-talk; that's how we talk to ourselves in our head. Given that people working within care have exceptionally high levels of self-criticism according to our research, then it's no surprise that a lot of care staff also have low confidence and self-esteem.

When we need to perform and get a good result it's critical that we have a level of confidence. If we talk to ourselves about what we should not do or what could go wrong then it creates an image of that very thing in our head. This is negative visualisation and as we've learned above, this can have a direct impact on how you perform.

Try this:

Say the words: **pink elephant**

Pause

Say it again: **pink elephant**

The chances are that you had an image pop into your mind's eye of a pink elephant.

Now try this: **Don't think about a pink elephant**

Can you do it? We can bet that elephant is still charging around in your mind!

The more you think about what not to do, or what not to think of, the more your mind visualises it. The solution is to simply tell yourself what you **do** want to see or how good you are going to be!

That's why, when working on the focusing technique, we use trigger words that enforce what we want to do such as 'calm' and 'focus'. If we used trigger words that say what not to do, such as: "Don't rush" then the chances are, we will rush.

Be positive and self encouraging at all times before, during and after your event. Use **DO** words, not **DON'T** words. Go on and indulge yourself in positive self-talk and tell yourself how good you're are going to be. It will pay off in the end.

AIR strategy – Bringing it together on the day of the event

A strategy we train people in so that they can get into the right state as they are about to perform is called the AIR Strategy. An acronym for: **Attention**, **Intention** and **Review**.

This is a simple strategy and system to create a consistent method that can help you get into the desired state time and time again. We developed this from sport psychology techniques that have now been adopted by many people from different sectors.

It's important that the technique is developed and practised in individual parts before bringing it all together. Obviously, this system can only be used in scenarios when you have the time to go through it, but with practice it can be done very quickly and even in under a minute.

A reminder: When we use the word perform, we don't necessarily mean a performance. We mean a situation where you want to be the best that you can be such as a team meeting, an inspection or visit from the local authority, or an important chat with a member of your team.

It works like this:

Stage 1 - Attention

Stage 1 takes place before you have entered the space in which you will perform.

Look and listen. Get yourself familiar with what is going on around the environment you will perform in. This creates an awareness and reduces the chance of shocks disrupting your state when performing.

Decision. Decide on what action you will take or review briefly what is pre-planned.

Assess state. Have a think about where your state is right now. Are you nervous or alternatively too relaxed? it's a case of look and feel within yourself and know if you have to either bring your state down from anxiousness or raise it up from drowsiness. Picture the state you need to be in and repeat in your head any opening line of your speech or first few seconds of the performance needed.

Stage 2 - Intention

This is when you are just about to perform and are in the final preparation. Sometimes it could be just a minute or so before the curtain goes up or you're about to begin.

Continue to build state using visualisation, controlled breathing and positive affirmations. Keep it simple. You don't want to fill your head with too much at this point.

Take a final breath and then simply let the performance happen. Trust yourself that you were rehearsed and in the right emotional state.

Other tips when performing are:

- Wiggle your toes in your shoes if you feel nervous, it helps with grounding you and stops you knees knocking!
- If something goes wrong then be ready to pause, re-set state, focus, relax and then carry on.

Stage 3 - Review

Results. After the performance and once the dust has settled consider if it was a good result or bad result, but always review the whole performance and do not let the result dictate your emotion when reviewing what happened. It can help to imagine watching the performance as a third party and commentating on what was awesome and what needed to be better.

Take the great elements and visualise yourself doing them again through your eyes as if you were actually doing them. This creates a powerful memory trace and helps you to repeat the performance again on another day.

Areas for development can be trickier because it's not good to be too self-critical, so review them as a third party and take advice from your new critic on what to do next time. Remember to use the affirmation of what you will do, not what you shouldn't do: "Next time be clear and concise" is a good example of what to say. Then simply re-run the development bits with a vision of doing them perfectly through your eyes as if you were doing them.

Summary

None of the state management techniques or the AIR stategy we have shared are of any use if you are not prepared to spend time practising them. Training your state is just like developing any other skill; you need to practice and invest in it and then you will have more capacity to manage your state when you need it.

Remember the more challenging the scenario ahead of you then the greater pressure you will potentially feel and the more state and mental capacity you will need to succeed. If you fail to manage your state during a performance you are likely to suffer the consequences and not get the result you are probably capable of.

We recommend practicing some of the state management techniques in less crucial scenarios, as preparation for the important ones. So, the next time you have a team meeting, try to run through some of the strategies beforehand. Ok, you may not get nervous or feel the need to manage your state for a team meeting, but you may still deliver a better meeting as a result.

By putting the practice in for non-critical scenarios, you'll find it easier to refer back to the strategies when you're next preparing for something that requires good state management, such as meeting your CQC inspector on their next visit.

Remember to help and develop others by sharing these strategies, or even get together as a team and practice them before an event that could require some state management.

Leadership styles

This could be the chapter that changes everything for you. We speak to so many people who have never really thought about their leadership or communication style and it can be quite transformational. If you're a new leader, learning this now will help you every step of the way to get the most out of your team, but we still meet plenty of experienced leaders who have never considered the different styles of leadership and how they can use them effectively.

There's a lot to cover so let's dive in.

We'll start with a definition of leadership:

> **Leadership** *is a process of social influence which maximises the efforts of others towards the achievement of a determined outcome.*

In other words, leadership stems from social influence, not authority or power. Leadership is never about YOU. It's about how you can influence people to get a desired result.

What's the best way to do that? It can depend on a few things, including the skill set of the people you're leading, their motivation levels and the situation at the time.

You will most likely have a natural leadership style that you are using right now and to find out what that is you can take the **Leadership Styles Questionnaire** which you can do in the book, over the page, or download and print a copy from the website: **www.careleadershandbook.co.uk** to fill in.

This questionnaire is based on the six leadership styles identified by Daniel Goleman (yes, he wrote the book on EQ too, he's a busy man!) and when you fill it in be sure to read the instructions carefully. It's important to fill it in as you are now, not how you would like to be, as that will give a true reflection of the style you are using the most right now. There's no right or wrong in this, so take it and then learn about the results in the following pages.

LEADERSHIP STYLES QUESTIONNAIRE

SCORING - READ THE FOLLOWING STATEMENTS AND AGAINST EACH STATEMENT ALLOCATE A SCORE:
"THIS IS ALWAYS TRUE OF ME": 5 POINTS
"THIS IS OFTEN TRUE OF ME": 3 POINTS
"THIS IS TRUE OF ME 50% OF THE TIME": 2 POINTS
"THIS IS LARGELY UNTRUE OF ME": 1 POINT
"THIS IS TOTALLY UNTRUE OF ME": 0 POINTS

1. MY TEAM TRUST ME IMPLICITLY ☐

2. I SPEND A LOT OF MY TIME GETTING BUY-IN TO IDEAS FROM MY TEAM MEMBERS ☐

3. I EXPECT PEOPLE TO DO AS THEY ARE TOLD, WITHOUT QUESTIONING MY MOTIVES ☐

4. I AM MORE INTERESTED IN SETTING LONG TERM GOALS THAN IN BEING INVOLVED IN DETAILED DAY TO DAY WORK ☐

5. I DELEGATE CHALLENGING ASSIGNMENTS, EVEN IF THEY WILL NOT BE ACCOMPLISHED QUICKLY ☐

6. I WOULD PREFER THAT TEAM MEMBERS BE HAPPY IN THEIR WORK THAN SPEND MY TIME CORRECTING EACH FAULT ☐

7. I EXEMPLIFY ALL THE STANDARDS THAT I EXPECT FROM MY TEAM ☐

8. I BELIEVE IN INVESTING TIME IN PEOPLE ☐

9. I TRANSLATE THE ORGANISATION'S STRATEGY INTO TERMS THAT THE TEAM CAN UNDERSTAND ☐

10. PEOPLE WHO DO NOT DO WHAT THEIR LEADERS TELL THEM DESERVE TO BE REPRIMANDED IMMEDIATELY ☐

11. I WORK HARD TO CREATE A STRONG SENSE OF BELONGING FOR ALL THE TEAM ☐

12. I THINK THAT WE CAN ALL GET A GOOD DEAL OF INSIGHT INTO AN ISSUE IF WE DISCUSS IT AS A TEAM ☐

13. WORK SHOULD BE VERY TASK-FOCUSED ☐

14. I SPEND TIME HELPING STAFF TO IDENTIFY THEIR OWN STRENGTHS AND AREAS FOR DEVELOPMENT ☐

15. I BELIEVE THAT DECISION-MAKING IN THE ORGANISATION SHOULD BE TOP DOWN ☐

16. I GIVE MY TEAM THE LEEWAY TO TAKE CALCULATED RISKS AND BE INNOVATIVE, ONCE I HAVE SET OUT THE DIRECTION THEY SHOULD TAKE ☐

17. I TRY TO SET A VISION AND GET STAFF TO COME ALONG WITH ME IN CREATING THAT VISION ☐

18. I AM NOT CONVINCED THE TEAM WILL WORK WITH INITIATIVE IF I DON'T DEMONSTRATE WHAT TO DO AND HOW TO DO IT ☐

LEADERSHIP STYLES QUESTIONNAIRE

SCORING - READ THE FOLLOWING STATEMENTS AND AGAINST EACH STATEMENT ALLOCATE A SCORE:
"THIS IS ALWAYS TRUE OF ME": 5 POINTS
"THIS IS OFTEN TRUE OF ME": 3 POINTS
"THIS IS TRUE OF ME 50% OF THE TIME": 2 POINTS
"THIS IS LARGELY UNTRUE OF ME": 1 POINT
"THIS IS TOTALLY UNTRUE OF ME": 0 POINTS

19. I WORK HARD TO ESTABLISH STRONG EMOTIONAL BONDS BETWEEN MYSELF AND MY TEAM ☐

28. I ENCOURAGE PEOPLE TO CREATE LONG-TERM DEVELOPMENT GOALS ☐

20. I GIVE PLENTIFUL INSTRUCTION AND FEEDBACK ☐

29. I GIVE MY TEAM MEMBERS REGULAR FEEDBACK ON THEIR PERFORMANCE ☐

21. I HOLD A LOT OF MEETINGS WITH MY TEAM TO ENSURE THAT THEY ARE HAPPY WITH THE WAY THAT THE TEAM IS WORKING ☐

30. I SET OUT WHERE I WANT THE TEAM TO GET TO, AND EXPECT THEM TO USE THEIR INITIATIVE IN GETTING THERE ☐

22. I KNOW WHAT IS BEST FOR MY TEAM AND EXPECT THEM TO DO WHAT I ASK ☐

31. I BELIEVE THAT WE CAN ALWAYS FIND WAYS TO DO THINGS BETTER AND FASTER ☐

23. COLLECTIVE DECISION-MAKING IS THE MOST EFFECTIVE FORM OF DECISION-MAKING ☐

32. I MAKE AGREEMENTS WITH MY TEAM ABOUT THEIR ROLES AND RESPONSIBILITIES AND ENACT DEVELOPMENT PLANS ☐

24. I IDENTIFY POOR PERFORMERS AND DEMAND MORE FROM THEM ☐

33. I GIVE THE TEAM FREEDOM TO ACHIEVE OUR GOALS ☐

25. IF PEOPLE DO NOT PERFORM WELL ENOUGH I BELIEVE THEY SHOULD BE QUICKLY REPLACED ☐

34. I BELIEVE IN LETTING THE TEAM HAVE A SAY IN THE WAY THE TEAM IS MANAGED ☐

26. IF I BELIEVED AN EXISTING SYSTEM WAS HAMPERING GOOD WORK, I WOULD HAVE NO HESITATION IN GETTING RID OF IT ☐

35. I HAVE GREAT SELF-CONTROL AND EXPECT TO USE MY INITIATIVE ALONE IN MANAGING OTHERS ☐

27. IN GIVING FEEDBACK I LOOK AT THE EXTENT TO WHICH A PERSON'S WORK HAS FURTHERED THE GROUP VISION ☐

36. I THINK THAT TEAM MEMBERS SHOULD HAVE A SAY IN SETTING GOALS AND OBJECTIVES ☐

LEADERSHIP STYLES QUESTIONNAIRE

ANALYSIS
TRANSFER YOUR SCORES FROM THE STATEMENTS IN THE QUESTIONNAIRE TO THE
APPROPRIATE STATEMENT NUMBERS IN THE GRID BELOW TO DETERMINE YOUR LEADERSHIP STYLES:

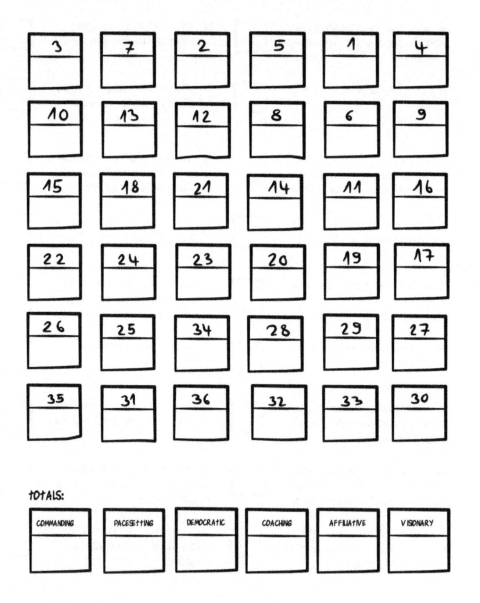

3	7	2	5	1	4
10	13	12	8	6	9
15	18	21	14	11	16
22	24	23	20	19	17
26	25	34	28	29	27
35	31	36	32	33	30

TOTALS:

COMMANDING	PACESETTING	DEMOCRATIC	COACHING	AFFILIATIVE	VISIONARY

The questionnaire will reveal the style you are using the most right now, and that may or may not be right for every situation. The best leaders will be able to change their style when required in order to get the best results from their team.

This might be a real revelation for you. Lots of people think they should adopt one particular style to be an effective leader, but we've all had a boss who's done that, and they've probably only had an impact on 10% of their staff. That's because a boss who says: "It's my way or the highway" will not get very far, especially with a team who is experienced and engaged. They will quickly get de-motivated if they are always being told what to do and the boss will find out that stamping their authority does not lead to desired results.

Have you experienced this type of boss? Sometimes our best lessons in leadership can be learning how not to lead. But let's flip that scenario and look at when it might be the right way...

If the building suddenly caught on fire, we wouldn't want the boss to be calling a meeting to discuss how to evacuate. In that situation we would want a boss who can command and instantly tell everyone what to do. In a crisis scenario, we would need our leader to go into a very "commanding" style of leadership that is clear and efficient and gets the job done.

So now we've got a bit of an idea about how leadership styles can change depending on the people or situation let's have a deeper look at the six different leadership styles.

The six leadership styles

Commanding

The commanding leader is all about gaining compliance from their people. They expect people to do what they tell them. This style works best when there is a crisis or with problem staff who have disciplinary issues, but it should be used sparingly as it can have a negative effect when used long-term. Staff will begin to feel like they are being denied the freedom to think and act for themselves if they are always being told what to do. This style will also have a negative impact on an experienced and motivated team.

Most likely to say – "Do what I tell you"

Pacesetting

The pacesetting leader will want to set high standards and emphasise accomplishing tasks. They will want things done their way, set timescales and may be referred to as slave drivers! This style can be useful when working towards a goal such as a CQC inspection where you might need to get everything in order within a set time frame, but staff could feel overwhelmed by the constant demand. They may find work is becoming too task focused and they are not trusted to use their own initiatives.

Most likely to say – "Do this by then and then do this by then"

Democratic

The democratic leader likes to get group consensus and is strong on collaboration, team leadership and communication. This style is great for getting input from staff or buy-in on ideas and can be useful when the leader is unsure on what to do and needs guidance. However, the democratic leader needs to be careful that this style doesn't result in endless, inconclusive meetings, and that they are not trying to get out of making decisions for themselves.

Most likely to say – "What do you think?"

Coaching

Coaching is the least used leadership style across the care sector but could be the most effective. A coaching leader will empathise the professional growth of their people and develop them. They will demonstrate empathy and self-awareness and be keen to improve performance and develop long-term strengths. The coaching leader needs to be careful not to waste their time with people who have no desire to learn or change and the style can take time to practice and see results from.

Most likely to say – "What does success look like?"

Affiliative

The affiliative leader likes to create harmony in the team. They will put people first and spend time building relationships with their staff. This style can be great when a team needs to be bonded or in stressful circumstances as the team will feel like their leader is one of them. An issue can arise when the team feel like their leader is not doing the job of guiding or setting direction. An affiliative leader should be careful to not let poor performance go unchecked or the team may start to run amok.

Most likely to say – "I'm here with you"

Visionary

The visionary leader emphasises the long-term goal and helps people to see the overall mission. They tend to have strong self-confidence and empathy for their staff. They can be great at driving change and this style is best used when change is needed or a clear direction needs to be set, such as when you're going for an improvement in your next CQC inspection. Visionary leaders should be cautious if they have an experienced team that their vision is not seen as out-of-touch or misjudged. They also need to be careful that the vision is clear and not changing direction every two minutes.

Most likely to say – "Come with me on this journey"

There are lots of famous speeches in history that you can read or watch and spot the leadership styles being used. In fact, you could probably lose a few hours on YouTube now going over some of the famous leader speeches of our time and thinking about why a certain style was used and what the impact of it was.

Probably the best example of a visionary leader and speech is Martin Luther King Jr's speech in 1963, calling for civil and economic rights and an end to racism in the United States. He repeatedly uses the words "I have a dream" and even holds his hand up in the air as thousands follow his hand and see his vision.

Another speech you will most likely recognise is when Winston Churchill addressed the nation in 1940 announcing that: "We shall fight them on the beaches, we shall never surrender" which is an example of mixing two different leadership styles; affiliative and commanding. By using the word 'we' he was making the British public feel that he was there with them, and everyone was in it together. But make no mistake that he was also commanding, there was no room for negotiation, he was telling the country what was going to happen.

Perhaps you can recall a powerful speech you've heard and can now think through what styles may have been used to communicate the message and influence those listening?

The words dictate the style

One really key point to understand is that the leadership style is dictated by the words you use, not the energy, volume or tone.

You can use the commanding style in a very loud and shouty way but also in a hushed and calm way. Think about when you might tell off your children. You might shout: "Go to your room!" at the top of your voice, but you could also say it in a calm, firm manner: "Go. To. Your. Room." Two very different tones, but the same commanding style. You are telling them what to do with no negotiation, discussion or input from them.

Bear that in mind as we continue through this chapter, as it can be tempting to think of certain styles, particularly the commanding style, as shouty when in fact it doesn't have to be.

Reviewing your own leadership style

Now that you have a clearer understanding of the different styles take a look at your own questionnaire results. Which style did you score the highest for? There is no right or wrong in this exercise, this should be clear by now, but it's important to reflect on the style that you are using the most and think about whether you are always applying it in the right way.

If your results show you are using the affiliative style the most right now, then think about the current performance of your team. Do they respect you as the leader or are you too 'in and amongst them' and not setting direction? We find that many people who are promoted to team leader adopt this affiliative style because they feel conscious that they've suddenly been promoted above their friends and don't want to annoy them by being too authoritative. The issue can come when their team mates then start to take advantage of the friendly style and standards start to drop. This can have a big impact on self-confidence so if that situation sounds familiar to you then there's steps you can take to manage it and become a great leader without losing your friends.

The other style we see often adopted by new leaders is the command style. This is so typical in a care setting because someone who is great at their job might get promoted to team leader and then feel that they have to exert some authority over the team to show that they've stepped up. It's also an easy style to default to, especially when you have a list of jobs a mile long. Telling people what to do can be an easy way to get things done quickly. However, over time we see this have a negative effect on the team, as they can become very frustrated by someone who was once 'one of them' now dictating everything they do.

Neither of these scenarios may be true of you, or at least not that dramatically, but potentially there may have been times you can recall where a different leadership style would have been more effective.

Typical scenarios to use different leadership styles

We thought we would throw out some ideas on how you might mix up your leadership styles in typical care scenarios:

Example 1. You've had your PIR, you know that the CQC inspection is impending, so it's time to gather your team and let them know what to expect from the day and instil some confidence in them. You could choose to use a visionary style of leadership here and share with them the vision you have of them all being perfectly competent and capable on inspection day and wowing the inspector with their enthusiasm. You could describe what it will look like when you receive the news that you've achieved outstanding and inspire them to believe that it's possible.

Example 2. The same scenario, but this time if you're feeling unprepared a pace-setting style of leadership could be useful. If you know you've got care plans to update and processes to get into place it may be worth getting task focused and being clear on the standards required. Remember this style of leadership shouldn't be used for the long-term, but could definitely help you in the run up to your inspection.

Example 3. You spot an unfamiliar car in the car park and know that this must be the CQC inspector... this is no time for a discussion! A command style of leadership may be necessary here to stop panic ensuing from the team. You may need to delegate very clear and direct orders to ensure the team are ready before the inspector walks through the door.

Example 4. A different scenario now. Every year you have a summer bbq and a few months before you start to plan the day. This might be a great time to adopt a democratic style of leadership and involve all of the team in the discussions and planning for the day. You may hear some great ideas from team members who don't normally speak up and it will enable you to get buy-in from the team.

Be aware that on the day of any type of event involving staff, clients, family members and potentially even children or pets could require a dramatic shift in your leadership style throughout the day! If plans are starting to go wrong and a thunderstorm begins you may have to go to the command-style to make sure everyone gets indoors without getting drenched. But if the sun is shining and everyone's having a great time it may be appropriate to adopt an affiliative style and get in amongst the team to help them relax and drive the feeling that you're one of them and down for some fun.

These examples should have started to get you thinking about how you can shift your leadership style to get the most out of your people and it's a good time to reflect on your results again and consider if you're using too much of one style or not enough of another.

> **Sophie says:** "People on our leadership academies often realise at this point that they've been sticking to one style, and how much more effective they could be as a leader if they adopt a different style, depending on the circumstances."

We are going to look a bit closer now as to how the situation can dictate the style of leadership you use.

Different ways to communicate

A good way to think about leadership styles is to think about how you communicate to your people. As we've mentioned the style is all about the words you use, but your team won't be listening and thinking: "Oh they are using a commanding style." They will be perceiving based on how you communicate the message.

Certain styles of leadership will generate a higher perceived level of ownership and responsibility for the person or people you are leading, while some of the styles will give very little perceived ownership.

This is why there is no single best style of leadership. You need to consider the skill set, knowledge and motivation levels of your people. And this means you might have to lead different people differently.

We sometimes get challenged on this when we teach it in our academies, and people have been known to say: "That's manipulation!" but remember, going back to the definition, that it's about social influence which maximises the efforts of others towards the achievement of a determined outcome. In order to maximise the efforts of others you may need to lead them in a different way to each other.

Let's explore how you might do this using the four communication styles.

Four ways to communicate

The four different ways to communicate are:

- **Tell**
- **Sell**
- **Discuss**
- **Empower**

You might already be able to see how the different leadership styles lend themselves to these, but it's important to look at the considerations for each.

Tell

If you have an inexperienced team on shift and know that there's a lot to cover in the day, then telling them what to do, how to do it and when it needs to be done may be the correct style. You could also be short on time and so this style ensures the message comes across clearly and concisely.

We see many care leaders using this style of communication every day within their environment. The problem can come when you have a team of experienced and competent care professionals who really don't need to be given the drill in this manner. If they know what they are doing, then constantly being "told" can demotivate them and damage culture.

> **Rob has a funny story about this:** "In a local village, the farmer has a meeting with his farm hands every morning around the kitchen table. He tells them where they're going to move the cows and how they're going to do it, and everything else that needs to be done that day. The issue is that his farm hands have been working the farm for nearly 40 years! They know exactly what the farmer is going to say, but he insists on telling them again every morning."

Sell

The sell style goes further than the tell style; it includes more of the "why" and an explanation as to why something is to be done to gain buy-in. You might need to communicate a decision that's been made by head office, but while no one can have control over that decision you still want them to feel enthused and excited about the decision.

Sometimes you may find yourself using the sell style when you need a favour from staff and there are various ways you can reward them for going the extra mile. The issue with this is that they can then start to expect a reward for actions that should be part of the job.

Discuss

Communicating through discussing things with your team is a great way to get them to collaborate, and if they feel they are involved in the decision making then they will have a greater ownership over the tasks you're discussing.

This is a good style to use with teams who are fairly motivated and with a good knowledge of the situation, as their input could be valuable.

Empower

Empower means to give someone the authority or power to do something. If you have an experienced, knowledgeable team who are highly motivated then the best thing you could do is to empower to make their own decisions.

By empowering your team they will feel valued as employees and feel a level of responsibility around the way the company is being run. It enables them to become self-leaders and means you can have a hands-off approach to be able to get on with your job.

Be aware that empowering people who are not knowledgeable and who do not have the right skills or motivation can be extremely detrimental. It could either crush their confidence if they don't feel ready for the responsibility and make a mistake, or with an unmotivated team you'll find that nothing will get done.

It may seem like there's a lot to consider before choosing your communication style with a team or with a single person, but by considering their skill set, knowledge and motivation you should be able to find the right style for the scenario.

Take a look at the graphic which shows how the leadership styles and communication styles fit with the level of ownership and responsibility that will be felt by the person or team. You may be able to plot your team members onto this graphic and see clearly what style is appropriate for which person, but bear in mind you may have to use several styles as the scenario presents.

COMMUNICATION STYLES

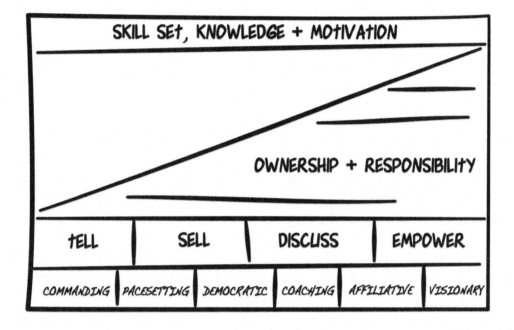

The end goal should be to move everyone across to the right hand side in terms of ownership and responsibility, and build a team of self-leaders that you can empower. It may just be that the skill set and knowledge are not quite there yet, but if the issue is motivation, then the next chapter will help you to address it.

Motivation

Motivation has been mentioned a number of times already in this book and a key to any company's success will be having a motivated team. Now it's time to delve deeper into motivation and how to drive it as a leader.

Motivation doesn't just have to be work related. We can be motivated by different things at work and in our personal life. There are various components related to motivation and we will explore each one within this section and how they interact to move us in certain directions. Let's look how the Oxford Dictionary defines the word before getting stuck into the how's and why's:

Motivation: *"A reason or reasons for acting or behaving in a particular way"*

We've noted before that the first six letters of motivation spell 'motive', and this suggests there will always be a reason for doing something.

Many people have a goal, such as: "I want to be an Outstanding rated manager" but fail to take enough action to achieve it. Perhaps you've seen this in someone else or in yourself? Whilst you may have a motive, the internal 'driver' that creates movement needs to be powerful enough in order for you to take that action.

The 'driver' is the emotional component. And if you look closely then another word that could be created from 'motivation' is 'motion' meaning movement.

So motivation requires a motive or reason and motion or movement, and the driver behind the movement is emotion.

Have a think for a moment about what motivates and moves you and how you motivate and move others around you. Earlier in the book we suggested that if you want movement in your people then you need to create emotion.

So if you want a big movement from your people then you need to find a way to create a lot of emotion in them.

We are going to look at how to do this now.

Motivational drivers

We can be motivated by both pain and pleasure, with pain typically influencing us to move away from something and pleasure influencing movement towards something. The degree of pain or pleasure will generally influence the pace and/or the quality of movement. You could also have both pain and pleasure working in tandem which you will have no doubt experienced or used yourself.

An example could be: "If you don't finish the care plans you will have to work late [pain], but if you get them finished you can go home early [pleasure]."

MOTIVATION

PAIN (PHYSICAL/MENTAL)	PLEASURE (PHYSICAL/MENTAL)
INTRINSIC (VALUES)	EXTRINSIC (MATERIALISTIC)

Other aspects that drive motivation include feelings and emotions that come from within us and link directly to our values such as pride, happiness and fulfilment or in contrast guilt, remorse and fear. We call these intrinsic drivers and they can be used to motivate us to move away from a negative emotional impact that causes pain or towards something that creates a positive emotional impact such as pride, which gives us pleasure.

Let's say that you go out of your way to help a client's family member for no other reason but that you wanted to. If you knew that there would be no additional benefit to helping them - no financial reward or time off in lieu and you did it purely because you wanted to and that it made you feel good inside then that is a great example of an intrinsic driver.

The opposite of an intrinsic driver would be an extrinsic driver, something you would do specifically for an external reward. This could be hitting a target purely to get a bonus. Looking at the motivation graphic you can see that this example combines motivation through extrinsic means and also pleasure. A different example combining extrinsic means and pain could be a threat that you would not receive the bonus unless you do something.

So it's important to look at the different combinations of:

- Intrinsic pleasure
- Intrinsic pain
- Extrinsic pleasure
- Extrinsic pain

Rob says: "When I was a kid, most of my school day extrinsic motivation was pain from teachers and featured a big cane and sore backside!"

How to motivate

It is possible for influence on motivation to come from all four aspects at the same time; pain, pleasure, extrinsic and intrinsic. But, let's not get overcomplicated and instead consider what combinations have the most powerful impact.

Believe it or not, pain has been proven to be far more effective in initially moving someone than pleasure. If you think about it, a quick threat of pain can make us react quickly. The downside is that pain can only be used as a motivator for so long because people either get used to it, so it becomes less effective or they find a way to avoid it. In a working environment, when pain is the primary motivator then people tend to quit.

Now think about what the leadership styles are in your working environment and how the management team motivate the staff. Is there any correlation in your staff turnover and how much 'pain' is being used?

Extrinsic pleasure such as a pay bonus, or a voucher will satisfy and motivate people so far but the problem with this is that people may get used to rewards and you may not always be able to give them one. Again this becomes less effective over time as they will come to expect rewards simply for doing their job and rewards are often not available in the care sector. This can then result in people not performing as you would want.

This leaves us to consider intrinsic pleasure as a combination for motivational influence. The reason this can be a great for long term means of moving people within the care sector is because it is driven by values.

What gets care professionals out of bed in the morning? It's often not extrinsic pleasure, as we know the care sector is not often highly paid. It's hopefully not based on any type of pain. Most people working in care, when asked, express a deep pride for doing what they do. It's the intrinsic pleasure that comes from doing what they do that gets them out of bed in the morning.

As a leader, if you can tap into your team's individual and group intrinsic pleasure drivers then you have the power to motivate them and move them to success.

So how do you find out what the true values-based motivators are and how can you shape and link them to what you want to get out of your team? Well, you can simply ask them! We know, bonkers isn't it, that we might just ask our people what really drives and moves them to do a good job or achieve a goal within work.

You can use this simple set of questions on your staff when you are searching their souls for the intrinsic values that motivate them, they are also ideal questions to ask during appraisals or supervisions, and even ask yourself:

- Why do you want to achieve it?
- Imagine you have done it. Now what does it look like?
- How does that make you feel?
- What do you think it says about you as a person for achieving that?
- And thinking about it, how does that make you feel?
- What do you think it makes those other people who have benefitted or who care about you feel knowing you have achieved this?
- And now knowing what you have made those close to you think and feel, how does it make you feel?

In this series of questions, you may have to double back and repeat questions again and again or dig deeper. You ultimately want to hear them tell you that they will be proud and happy or words to that effect. Don't let them off with just: "I will feel good", go deeper into the emotions. You may also get some responses about extrinsic value areas such as: "I will get a pay rise" and that's fine but make sure you bring it back to the intrinsic values.

Once you know what it is that drives them, and you have linked it to very deep and meaningful values and loved ones they will likely be very motivated to achieve and complete the goal or job well. If they don't you can simply remind them of the conversation and the reason why they should be performing better, and take them back to their intrinsic values of pride and happiness that they expressed to you before.

If you've ever experienced this for yourself, having someone remind you of your intrinsic values when you're not working to your potential will be the most painful and toughest conversation you will have in a long time!

It's all very well us sharing about how to motivate people, but it might not be the right approach for everyone and in some cases might not be necessary. With the right people, you'll have a profound effect and see results, but we don't want you to waste time on people if it's not the right approach right now.

Thinking back to some of the leadership and communication styles we shared earlier, you may now be thinking about who you can motivate in your team and who you may struggle with. We mentioned that you could plot your team into a chart to understand which approach will work best, and in the next section we are going to show you a simple exercise to help you do just that.

The Skill Will Matrix

It would be an ideal workplace if you as a leader could simply empower your staff to complete tasks and duties without worrying whether the job will get done and to the standard you require. In reality, you may have some staff who you cannot empower because of their inexperience, or you may even have some who are lazy. What's interesting is these tend to be the people who take up most of your time when you could be doing other things.

Empowerment has been a buzz word for a long time in business and we often hear leaders talking about how: "We must empower everyone." Well, that would be ideal, but only if they are ready to be empowered.

If someone is lazy and you empower them then don't be surprised when you go to check and the task is not complete. Likewise, if a person is unskilled and they are empowered then regardless of their willingness and motivation they could fail to complete the task. This could also have a negative impact on their confidence and de-motivate them to try again.

So, the only time you should be fully empowering staff is if they are motivated and skilled enough. If they are not, then we should consider a different or modified approach.

We have emphasised throughout this book that leaders need to be flexible in their approach and style of communication. Sometimes it will be appropriate to be direct and tell, and on other occasions you may be able to empower or coach your staff. The Skill Will Matrix is a simple tool that helps you to consider which approach you might take to get the best out of the different people that work for you.

In the section about communication styles we laid out when it might be appropriate to use either tell, sell, discuss or empower and the Skill Will Matrix links these styles to the persons readiness to work. You can download and print a Skill Will Matrix template from the website: **www.careleadershandbook.co.uk**

SKILL WILL MATRIX

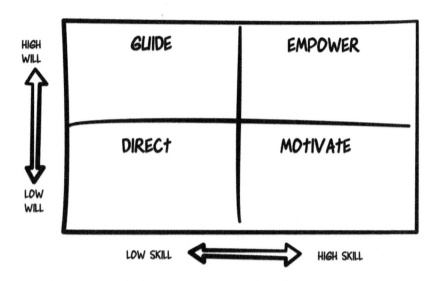

To use the Matrix simply have a staff member in mind and think about to what extent they are motivated (their will power) and also how skilled they are. Depending where they are in these two separate areas you simply plot them on the chart - along the vertical for will and horizontal for skill.

Example – you could have a new staff member who lacks skill but is highly motivated, so they will feature in the top left box.

Or, perhaps you have someone highly skilled but who lacks motivation, such as a staff member who has been doing the job for years, knows everything there is to know, but lacks any drive or motivation. This person would feature in the bottom right of the matrix.

To get more accurate with this you can section the matrix into a grid 0-10 on both the vertical and horizontal.

Example - Harry your new carer may score 3/10 on skill but 9/10 on will and motivation and therefore plot him on the intersection of these scores up in the top left box. You can repeat this for the entire team or sit in a small management group to do it together. It's worth considering where you sit in the matrix too.

Now you have plotted staff on the matrix you should reflect and consider how you communicate to them when delegating tasks and more importantly how effective they are at completing those tasks. If the tasks are not getting done to time and standard required then recognise that you are partly to blame. You are the leader and therefore have ultimate responsibility and that includes ownership of that responsibility.

We know it would be fantastic if every time you give out a task and job it was completed but we also know it doesn't always happen like that, so let's look at how adapting your style to accommodate for where people sit on the matrix could help you get more from them.

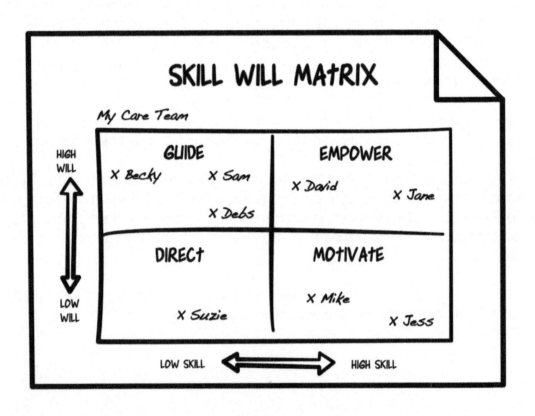

Typical examples you may relate to

Chris is a care professional who is highly skilled but lacking will power and motivation. How could you communicate and manage Chris so that ultimately you could empower him?

It's going to come down to creating the passion and excitement in him to be motivated for work so that he utilises his skills and can be trusted to simply get on with work without the need for supervision.

Strategies to motivate skilled staff (not all will be appropriate):

- Ask them what would motivate and excite them in their work.
- Use your coaching skills (covered in the next chapter) with them and search for the purpose that they get from working in care and use this as an emotional lever.
- Offer additional responsibilities if they need challenge to stay motivated.
- Make them a mentor and emphasise that they are a role model.
- Create reward incentives or consequence of not performing. (Use sparingly)

Consider the benefits of finding the motivation from within Chris. It will free up your time as a leader to do the things you should be doing. The team will have a much better relationship if they're all as equally motivated and above all your clients will receive better care.

Sarah is a care professional who is new in the role and very motivated (high will power) but because she is new and inexperienced, she lacks competence (low skill).

We have heard managers say to the Sarah's of this world: "Don't run before you can walk" and this can stamp out all the drive and motivation in them.

The last thing you should do as a leader is stifle their enthusiasm. In such situations you simply need to find out what knowledge and skills are required by Sarah and guide her along a pathway of development at the same time as maintaining her will/motivation. This will also build her confidence as she learns. It may not be long before Sarah is highly skilled and motivated and ready to be empowered. Sarah is ideal to be coached and guided.

Tiffany is a care professional who is not skillful and she also lacks motivation. She often lets you down and you constantly need to check on her work. Tiffany takes a lot of your time and effort to manage. There are a few considerations here. Firstly, there was a hiring mistake (more on hiring later) and secondly, has she used up all of her excuses and is it time to help her to find employment elsewhere?

If you choose to keep Tiffany then you need to be very focussed on how to get the best performance from her. Essentially, for now, she needs **telling**! Tiffany should definitely not be empowered.

Johnny is a care professional who is highly skilled and very motivated. He is the sort of guy you just know will deliver care to he highest standard and never let you, the team or the clients down. Johnny is an ideal member of staff who you should empower.

If you use a tell and command style approach with Johnny then he will feel under-valued and not trusted. He then might slip down into the bottom right hand box and become an unmotivated but skilled carer or worse he could leave and go somewhere where he will feel appreciated and challenged. So, what can you do with Johnny to keep him motivated and skilled? You need to challenge him so that he is excited and this could be with strategies such as:

- Reward such as promotion or pathway to promotion, but also consider his values and how he is motivated by praise and recognition.
- Up-skilling with additional training.

- Additional challenging tasks and responsibilities - not just volume but quality challenges.

Now is a good time to reflect on the staff you have plotted on the skill will matrix and consider how you actually manage and communicate with them and start to adjust your approach if needed. Your aim is to move as many staff members into the top right corner as possible. This will create a highly efficient and engaged team; the sort that Outstanding care companies have.

Coaching

Up until now you've learned about emotional intelligence, you've learned how to manage your state under pressure, you've learned about your leadership style and how to communicate and motivate. Now we are going to focus exclusively on the coaching style of leadership, and this will be a chunky chapter of this book. Coaching will help you to bring a lot of what you've learned so far together.

Leadership and coaching are inextricably linked, so we knew we had to cover coaching in great detail as it's one of the most powerful strategies you will learn that will support you to lead your team.

As we've already mentioned, coaching is one of the least used but most effective leadership styles so it's worth taking a deeper dive in to it. If coaching was widely adopted in the care environment it would have a powerful impact on the sector as it's especially good for shaping culture and developing people.

COACHING PROCESS

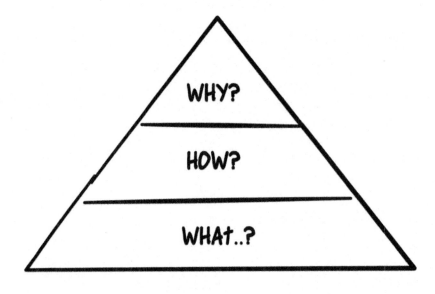

Discovering the **what**, the **how** and the **why** is the fundamental core of coaching. Always have those three words in the back of your mind when embarking on a coaching session.

Earlier, when we explored leadership styles, we established that words are a key factor in determining the style used. For coaching, the words should always be 'asking' and 'exploring' questions.

We have found, working with care companies, that many care leaders **think** they coach when in fact they **tell** and **direct** and so this, by definition is not coaching. We think that perhaps the reason why care leaders' often default to the 'tell' style of communication is because they are natural 'fixers and helpers' and want to help because they can. Telling people what to do is also a quicker method of getting a result and time can be a very precious commodity within the care environment.

However, when you look below at some of the philosophy and ethos of coaching you will see that we often miss an opportunity to fully develop people because we take over the problem and solution ourselves and fail to coach. If we applied more coaching then it would help drive ownership of learning and development for the person being coached and this has lots of other benefits. It can help to create empathy between yourself and the person you coach, it gives you an ability to empower them, and it gives them a sense of fulfilment and that they are valued by you and the company.

Coaching versus mentoring

A lot has been written regarding the differences between coaching and mentoring and you will probably find dozens of different comparisons if you look online, so let's keep it simple here and give some examples.

A coach is able to work with anyone, even if they don't have experience in their field of work, because the asking style required for coaching creates a situation where the person being coached finds the development pathway for themselves.

A mentor, however, needs to have a level of understanding about the field of work so that they can be more direct and give advice and suggestions.

For instance, we could coach a doctor to become a better doctor, but we could not mentor the doctor because we lack the medical skills and knowledge. From a mentoring perspective an experienced doctor could mentor another less capable doctor but could not mentor a bricklayer, unless of course they had great bricklaying ability too!

It is also possible that an experienced care leader could coach and mentor a less capable care professional providing of course they had adequate coaching ability and knew how to mentor.

Read and explore the suggestions in this chapter and you will be well on your way with coaching. Get this right and you will create a very resilient and happy team who will surpass your expectations of performance.

The principles of coaching

The key principle of coaching is to provide opportunities for others to learn about their own performance, their limitations and their solutions. It is crucial that the coach leader creates a climate for learning.

With this in mind think about your company and consider if it has a culture that will support coaching and learning. The company needs to have people who are willing and want to learn or have a desire to be more efficient and motivated to do a great job.

The main barrier to this is often what we can only describe as the 'old farts' who do the bare minimum and don't want to change.

Sophie says: "We couldn't think of a better way to phrase this! Perhaps 'can't change, won't change ones' would be another description, but either way we are sure you know who we mean!"

You will need to either find a way to change them or, dare we say it, support them to find gainful employment elsewhere! We know staffing can be a struggle in care, but sometimes it's better to be mercenary and cut loose the few that are holding the rest of the company and the culture back.

If you think the culture on the whole in your company is an issue or that a few people will be a challenge then review the chapter later in the book on developing culture. If the culture is poor then ultimately your coaching efforts might be less effective than you had hoped.

People get the best results from coaching in a place where it is safe to disclose information and share ideas that, perhaps, have never been disclosed before. Trust must be built, so see over the page the principles of coaching which you can download from the website: **www.careleadershandbook.co.uk** and pin up on a notice board in your office if you wish:

PRINCIPLES OF COACHING

- Ownership of goals and aspirations are owned by the coachee

- Never take responsibility for the coachee's results - they own their goal

- Stay non-judgement and non-critical. Stay positive

- Believe the coachee has the answers within them and will be able to find the solution for themselves

- Break down big goals into manageable steps

- Have a genuine willingness to learn

- Respect confidentiality

- Build and maintain self-esteem in the coachee

- Challenge and move the coachee beyond their comfort zone

- Believe that there are always solutions to be found

- Pay attention to recognising and pointing out strengths in the coachee

- Believe that self-knowledge improves performance

A change of thinking

As mentioned earlier it's sometimes hard for great care leaders to excel as a coach as they often want to be the fixer of the problems, so it may need a fundamental change of how you, as a care leader think, in order to resist the urge to tell rather than ask.

A coach needs to drop their own agenda to resolve other people's problems and develop a more open-minded approach, resisting the temptation to tell and guide individuals towards solutions.

Coaching is about a principled, trustworthy and honest approach to support people in finding their own solutions. A coach rarely offers their own advice, unless of course they are taking a coach and mentor approach. This is fine but remember it detracts the ownership from the coachee and is not an approach we are going to focus on here.

When coaches give advice or guidance, they steal away from the coachee a level of understanding around the process. If the coachee does not understand the process, then they return again for advice. Coach them, and then they find the answers and the process to use next time.

Good coaches foster the belief in their people that if they think an issue or problem through, then they will know the next step in resolving it; all they need to do is to take action and follow their own solution, which will lead to improvement.

Ask yourself these questions. Do you:

- Complete other people's sentences in your head before they have finished?
- Move on in your mind to the solution you would choose for the person?
- Use closed questions? (These are questions that can only be answered with a yes or a no)
- Use leading questions to guide others to a specific solution that you have identified?

- Almost instantly believe that you know the answer they are looking for?
- Make up your mind on the way to resolve a problem or enhance performance and push that idea?
- Become angry if your solutions for others are rejected?
- Find that your ideas are not implemented, then the same individual returns with other problems for you to resolve?
- Secretly acknowledge that you don't have the answers?

If any of the above apply to you, then coaching could be a way of relieving frustrations, dissipating anger and taking the pressure off of yourself to come up with the answer.

Coaches should be curious, ask questions and support students to learn about their situation fully. Coaches are more than problem-solvers, they encourage others to understand their beliefs and amend their behaviours to allow optimum performance.

Alfred Korzybski in 1933 explained the concept that: "the map is not the territory". In other words, what one person experiences in a situation is not necessarily how others experience it and vice versa.

When did you last experience something that seemed very different to another person? Have you ever had an interaction with a client and another member of staff and then your reflections on that interaction have been different to your team member? This is precisely why asking, rather than telling, allows you to understand the other persons 'map of the world' and develop a deep empathy with the way they see things.

We're going to explore how you can unlock someone's map of the world next. But to be clear about what coaching can do for you as a leader and for your team:

Coaching will allow you to promote independent thinking in others and if your people can become resilient and good at self-solving then you will be on the way to empowering them and reducing how much wasted time you spend fixing people issues in your company.

How to coach

Now that we've gone through the concept and benefits of coaching it is time to put it into practice. We recommend finding someone in your team who you feel comfortable with who is open to being coached. Perhaps someone who is struggling with a certain aspect of the job or has had an incident at work. You could even try this with a friend or member of your family.

Throughout this section we will refer to you as the **coach** and the person you are coaching as the **coachee**.

It is important to contract the session right at the beginning and ensure both yourself and the person you are coaching are fully aware and happy to proceed. By contract, we don't mean you need to physically sign a contract. We just mean that before you start, you need to have a quick conversation to agree terms. It helps you both know you're on the same page before you start.

Contract the session and ensure you:

- Share expectations of the session including confidentiality, honesty and integrity.
- Agree to both commit to the coaching session.
- Discuss the length of the session.
- Agree if and how the session will be recorded. Will you write notes or email a summary of the session?

Sophie says: "*Agreeing how much time you have is crucial! You don't want to spend half an hour going through the coaching process and then get cut short. Coaching can be done over a long cup of coffee, but it can also happen very quickly on-the-go, so agree the time you have before you start.*"

Once you have contracted the session the coaching process is a three-stage approach to help a person improve their own performance.

It begins with you raising the coachee's **awareness** about themselves and what they are capable of. In doing so, your aim is to **generate responsibility** in the coachee, so that they can decide for themselves what they want and what they must do in order to get it. By raising awareness and generating responsibility in this way, your final aim is to **facilitate** and empower a person to improve their performance and achieve more under their own terms.

COACHING PROCESS

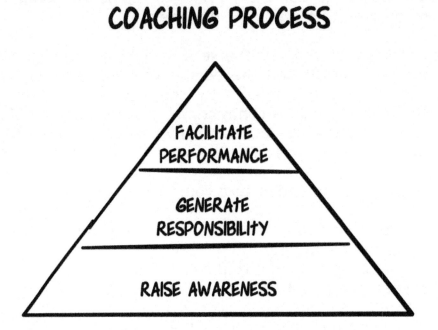

FACILITATE
PERFORMANCE

GENERATE
RESPONSIBILITY

RAISE AWARENESS

One final point is that coaching doesn't have to be a formal, sit-down conversation in an office. You want to get the best out of the coachee and they may feel more comfortable in a local café or you may even decide that a walk around the garden creates the ideal environment for them to relax.

Raising Awareness

One of the first things to do when coaching is to raise awareness. It seems simple but it takes a subtle style of questioning to do it effectively. Essentially, it's about getting the person to become conscious of themselves and what they want to achieve. It will also raise your attention to their thoughts and feelings, help with developing empathy and enable you to see their 'map of the world'.

Often, the information a person needs in order to solve the problem and improve their performance is available to them – they just don't know it. This could be because they are distracted by things such as stress and negativity or could be because they lack the self-confidence to work things out for themselves.

Throughout this book we cover barriers to performance, resilience and self-leadership and these are often the classic factors that prevent people from moving forward. You will find that many have never taken the time to sit down and reflect upon what it is that is important to them and what it is that they want to achieve.

A caution:

Be prepared for tears on occasion when you coach, as these moments can be very emotional if the discussion goes into a deep personal spot. You would be surprised how some seemingly simple, superficial goals sometimes have a much deeper purpose behind them.

When you raise someone's awareness to their potential, and they feel they are being understood, emotion can rise to the surface, so have the tissues ready! We are certainly not saying you should be aiming to make people cry in your coaching sessions, but any time that emotions are explored, there is always the potential for tears.

There are two types of awareness that the coach needs to raise. Firstly, there is general awareness. General awareness is about the 'bigger picture'; what is happening around that person. Whenever a person has a problem or wants to achieve something, it normally involves other people, whether in work or in their personal life. We sometimes call this the 'outside world'. The coach therefore needs the coachee to reflect upon their knowledge and beliefs about these things, for instance what effect other people have on them and what effect they have on other people.

Then there is self-awareness. Whilst general awareness is about what is happening around a person, self-awareness is about what is happening within them, their 'self-world' as we sometimes say. Self-awareness is about considering why they think, feel and act the way they do, like in the performance spiral we looked at earlier in the book. Whilst a person may already be aware of these things subconsciously, the role of the coach is to make them consciously aware of them too.

Example: Let's say Mel comes to you because she wants a promotion to team leader. By raising her awareness you're helping her to understand where she is now in terms of performance, attendance and what her capability is. You would also want her to be aware of what the benefits of the promotion would be, but also, anything that could be a negative about the promotion, such as longer hours or more paperwork, which she may not have considered.

While you are speaking with Mel about her ambitions, ensure that you use **effective questioning** to uncover the answers from her.

Generate Responsibility

When a person truly accepts or takes responsibility for their thoughts, feelings and actions, their commitment rises and their performance improves even if it's a boring or an unpleasant task. This is the main reason why ownership has such an impact on performance and doing a good job.

When a person is **told** to take responsibility or is placed in a situation where they are expected to take responsibility but do not fully accept it, their performance, invariably, does not improve. Whilst a person may perform and get through the task because they have to, they certainly won't aspire to the highest of standards. You may have seen this within your own company?

Awareness is one of the cornerstones of responsibility because it brings that person a sense of certainty about themselves, other people and the world in which they live. The coachee must come to realise that if anyone is going to make things happen, it has got to be themselves. The other cornerstone of responsibility is choice.

When a person is told to do something and they feel that they have no choice in the matter, their lack of ownership means that they do not feel responsible. This is a double-edged sword because if the person fails in whatever they have been told to do, they will end up blaming the person who told them what to do; and haven't we all blamed the boss in the past for something we had no choice in doing?

Even if the person succeeds in whatever they have been told to do, they may feel that success wasn't achieved through their own efforts or choice. A leader coach therefore needs to ensure that the person feels that they are in control of what they want to achieve and how they are going to get it. The coachee must feel that they have complete ownership of the whole coaching process.

In this way, awareness and choice lead to responsibility, then the awareness and responsibility leads to performance. The role of the coach is to help the person through this process to the point whereby they have both. The above points will also relate to a simple task and not just the big goals that someone has. If you can adopt a coaching style of communication as you lead your team you will see general levels of responsibility and commitment improve all around you.

Example: Now Mel is aware of what going for the promotion will entail, you should be able to generate some responsibility from within her about what she needs to do to achieve the promotion. She may need to speak to someone who is already a team leader to get some advice, or she may need to study and pass a few exams. As the coach, you want to know that she is prepared to do the things she needs to in order to gain the promotion, it won't just be handed to her on a plate.

You need to be **actively listening** while Mel tells you what she's going to do, in order to establish whether she is really going to take the appropriate steps. Don't just listen with your ears, check her body language and enthusiasm to gauge if she is committed.

Facilitate Performance

This is simply helping someone to commit and achieve what they have set out to do and in coaching terms it is described as facilitating performance.

Whilst raising awareness and generating responsibility are the key aims of coaching, it's also critical that the coachee has a high self-image, feels good about their ability and is up for it!

Self-image can have a real impact on this and self-image is what you see in the mirror or your perception of yourself in a given scenario. It's possible for your self-image to change and go higher or lower, depending on the scenario.

Rob says: "If I had to sing a karaoke song in public my self-image might be low as I'm pretty tone deaf, but if I had to talk to someone about leadership, then my self-image would hopefully be high."

The problem when the coachee is in low self-image and subsequently has negative feelings is that they tend not to be able to tap into their motivational drivers. Likewise, when a person has a low self-image, they are unlikely to accept responsibility preferring instead to not bother doing something, blame everyone but themselves or simply wallow in self-pity.

Therefore, to facilitate performance you may need to use a variety of skills and techniques. These could be goal setting exercises or if confidence is an issue you may have to use certain strategies and techniques to get them over that hurdle before they can move forward effectively. We are going to cover all of this later in the book.

When a person has a high self-image their subconscious mind remains open and receptive to the things they want to achieve. They not only accept responsibility – they will actively seek it! A coach must make a conscious effort to be aware of a person's self-image throughout the coaching process.

A coach must try to raise self-image and maintain it at a high level during the initial stages of the coaching relationship and in simple terms, make people feel good and positive about themselves. It's not enough to just tell someone to be positive it doesn't work like that. You will need to use effective questioning to make the person feel good and in high self-image and that way they take ownership and get results.

Example: As the coach, you want Mel to feel like she can achieve this promotion, so be sure to give her encouragement and let her know how you can support her with the process. The goal setting exercise later in this book may be useful for her and will let you put your coaching skills into practice.

Make sure you are giving **empathic responses** during this part of the conversation. If you show doubt about her ability to achieve it then you could influence her to not take the next steps to her goal.

Coaching Skills

As we've eluded to in the example running through this chapter, the skills you need to deploy as a coach are **effective questioning, active listening** and an **empathic response**.

These skills are not easy to master, and it can be quite frustrating when you're first getting started, but remember as you work through the process that:

- In order to raise awareness, you need to ask effective questions
- You should actively listen to understand if you have generated responsibility
- An empathic response is required in order to facilitate performance.

COACHING SKILLS

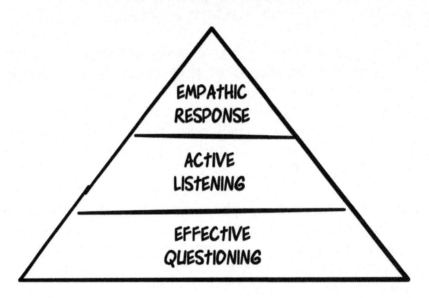

We know that this is a big chapter with a lot to think about. We felt it was important to explain the entire process and the science behind coaching.

Everything moving forward in this section of the book will allow you to practice coaching. Every exercise can be done using a coaching style of leadership and we will emphasise this throughout the next few chapters.

To start, we have a fun, practical and interesting exercise with a clear process to help you practice your coaching skills.

Wheel of performance

It's time for a practical exercise to get you started using your coaching skills.

We love using this model and we've found that care managers have had great success using this with their teams. It will really test your resistance to 'tell' as it's all about asking questions, and it will help build your confidence to tackle some of the other models we will show you later in the book.

If you're a manager with line managers below you then this can be useful to teach them and then it can be cascaded down into the home or company so that everyone has been through the experience of creating a wheel with a coach.

You may have seen a wheel of life before or completed one; lots of life coaches use it as a starting point when they first start working with someone to get a better idea of where they are happy and where they need development.

Used in your care company it will give you as the leader a really good idea of where your team are and can really help with any supervision conversations going forward or appraisals. It's also visual which makes for great evidence for your well-led KLOE for CQC.

You may want to complete a wheel for yourself first, to get comfortable with the steps. When you're ready, find someone willing to participate, find somewhere quiet and remember to contract the session as we explained in the chapter on coaching.

How to complete the wheel with a member of your team

We're going to go through the steps using an example:

 Let's say Lauren has been with the company for six months and has passed her probation and you think this is a good time for her to reflect on how she's doing. You've got to know her and think she may need improvement in some areas but now is a really good time to understand from Lauren's perception where she is now and where there she may need development.

Start the session by building rapport and contracting the session.

Explain the exercise to Lauren and why you're doing it.

 Start by drawing the wheel or print a copy from our website: **www.careleadershandbook.co.uk** and you might want to print the list of the descriptors to help her decide which ones to add to her wheel.

WHEEL OF PERFORMANCE

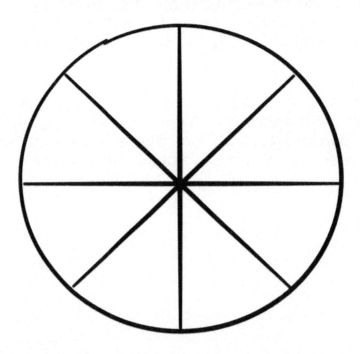

Have Lauren look at the list and think about her current role and what makes up her current role. Have her select 8 descriptors to make up the spokes of the wheel. It's up to Lauren whether she wants to fill this in herself, or she might want to sit back and let you do it. Let her decide.

LISt OF DESCRIPtORS

ACCOUNTABILITY	tIME MANAGEMENt	ACtIVE
CARING	ENTHUSIASM	KNOWLEDGE AND SKILLS
LEADING	SENSITIVITY	ENERGY
tEAMWORK	PATIENCE	RESPECt
COMMUNICATION	PROFESSIONALISM	PUNCtUALITY
INITIATIVE	HONESTY	HUMOUR
SUPPORTING	SELF MOTIVATION	DEPENDABLE
WELLBEING	ADAPTABILITY	WORK EtHIC
COOKING	ORGANISED	CREATIVE

Add the 8 descriptors around the wheel – and we recommend no more than 8. If you're pushed for time you might even want to start with just 4.

Now take each descriptor one by one. Let's say Lauren has 'professionalism' as one of her spokes. Your job as the coach is to ask her first what a ten out of ten for professionalism would look like for her. As she starts speaking, listen to the words she's using and make sure she's describing what a ten out of ten **would** be, not where she feels she is now. This is very important as it helps to benchmark what a perfect score would be.

Once she's described everything that she believes would be a ten out of ten for professionalism ask her to reflect where she would score herself right now. She should find this relatively easy now she has a comparable.

You may or may not agree with Lauren's score, but it's important to stay neutral at this stage – remember coaching is about asking questions, not telling! This is also a reflection of Lauren's 'map of the world' and what she thinks. Gently challenge Lauren on her score, ask her why she has given herself that score, and in light of how she has described a ten, does that score seem fair? If you feel she has been particularly tough or generous to herself you may want to give some real-life examples that might help her adjust it if needed, but make sure the final decision comes from her. Make a note of the number, fill in the spoke of the wheel to the correct level and move on to the next spoke and repeat the steps.

This exercise can get tricky if the participant does not fully describe what a ten out of ten is first. If there is no benchmark, then how can they score themselves? Make sure they've described what constitutes a perfect score before you let them score themselves, it will make it much easier for you to challenge their score!

Once the wheel is complete both sit back and look at the whole wheel. What stands out to you? Is it fairly balanced or if this wheel was on the road would it be a bumpy ride? As you've been going through the exercise you'll already have some idea as to whether Lauren's perception of herself matches up to your own opinion, but now you will clearly see if there are any areas she feels underconfident or unskilled in, or just needs to improve.

There may be something obvious you can tackle as a next stage right away, or you may want to schedule a follow up to go through some of the areas she's not scored herself as well in. If Lauren's given herself a low score for knowledge and skills for example, you might be able to discuss right away what steps you can take to improve that score. Alternatively this may make a good pre-appraisal exercise, giving you both some time to go away and think before the appraisal about where Lauren can develop and how to do that.

Sophie says: *"Watch out for people who say a ten out of ten in any area is unachievable. Besides making for a depressing looking wheel, it's not the point of the exercise to make a ten out of ten unachievable! A ten out of ten should be something that is achievable within their role so make sure when they describe it that they are not referencing the impossible!"*

The completed wheel may look something like this:

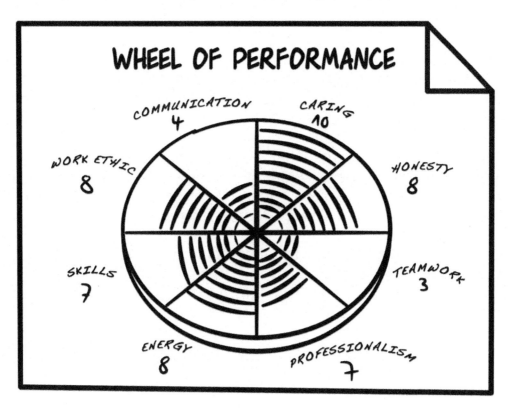

So just to capture those steps again:

1. Define the spokes of the wheel
2. Describe what a 10/10 would look like
3. Rate and score
4. Challenge the score and adjust if needed

What next

Make sure you both have a copy of the wheel and now you can move on to the rest of your team. Imagine what an insight into their own perceptions you're going to have when you have completed wheels for everyone. We've seen managers have these pinned up on a noticeboard (you can remove the names if you like) and this has been a colourful reminder of where the team may collectively need development. Use this information as a starting point for your supervision conversations and move on to use one of our other models, such as the GROW model (coming up) for anyone who has goals to set off the back of this exercise.

Reflect on yourself and how you did in your first coaching exercise. Did you stick to the time allocated? Did you resist the urge to 'tell' the answers or share your own perception? It can feel like a hard and slow process but by doing so you'll be getting the best out of your staff and encouraging them to think for themselves. It's exactly what we talked about earlier – you're raising their awareness, helping to generate responsibility and once you have a completed set of wheels you may be able to see clearly how you can facilitate great performance.

Later, we will look at how to use this exercise with an entire team to create 'team wheel's which can be used to develop the company culture. It may be useful to come back to this chapter and refresh yourself on the process when you get there.

Goal setting

If you've tried the wheel in the previous chapter, then a goal setting exercise may be the natural next step. Again, it provides a framework for you to comfortably practice your coaching skills.

The development of staff is a continuous challenge within the care sector, so we have included a simple and well-proven goal setting model called the GROW model that can help staff unlock dreams and goals and really keep them on a performance track.

It can be used with individuals or with groups and can be formal, as part of an appraisal process or even just as and when, depending on the scenario. The GROW model is best used with a coaching style of leadership and completing the exercise with members of your team is a great way for you to pick up from the previous chapters and practice coaching.

When you first have a go at this, try to find someone in your team who you are comfortable with, who has a goal in mind. It could be passing an exam, improving their computer skills or getting a promotion. All of these are tangible goals you can coach them to achieve using this model. You could even try this at home with your children who are hoping to pass exams or achieve something in their lives!

Introduction to the GROW model

In this section we will refer to you as the 'coach' and your colleague the 'coachee'.

You should use an effective questioning style, rather than a 'tell' style in order to:

- Raise the coachee's awareness to their development needs and the depth of the goal.
- Create enthusiasm in the coachee to be coached.
- Help them take ownership of their own learning.
- Help them set their own goals.
- Help them make realistic action plans.

- Help them find solutions and answers for themselves.
- Build their commitment to implementing their plans and reach their goals.
- Support them in applying and refining further what they have learnt.

To ensure a relevant focus and clear outcomes, the GROW model has a four-step agenda that covers:

- **Goal**
- **Reality**
- **Options**
- **Will**

When using these questions use whatever words fit your natural style and language and the context of your care environment: there is no need to repeat the exact wording in the checklist, just have the words in your mind to keep you on track.

The words can also be used at the start of a coaching session, to set the goal and clarify expectations during the session itself to draw out the learning, or after a session to summarise and consolidate the learning.

You do not need to use every one of these questions listed in every coaching session. Whilst a questioning approach is usually the most effective, there will be times when the coachee does want some direction, information or feedback from you, in which case excessive questioning may simply irritate or frustrate them. Bear in mind that if you do begin to give feedback or information then you are drifting into more of a guided mentor style and be sure you are competent and have the subject knowledge to direct whoever you are working with.

When we've worked with care professionals and taught them this framework around goal setting, they have found the hardest part was trying not to offer solutions and opinion. The desire will always be there to simply tell the coachee what you think, especially if you can see the answers for yourself. Resist this as much as you can, as it will strengthen your ability as a coach if you can stick to asking effective questions as much as possible.

How to take someone through the GROW model

Let's say that you are about to coach a member of your team who wants to pass an exam in the next few months. You've got a bit of time with them and are able to find a quiet room to take them through the GROW model.

Begin by contracting the session as we shared earlier, so that you know how much time you have and expectations are shared.

If you're able to have a pen and paper to hand, start by drawing the GROW model out on a piece of A4 or download a copy from **www.careleadershandbook.co.uk** and print. Explain that you're going to look at this goal with them and work through how they might achieve it.

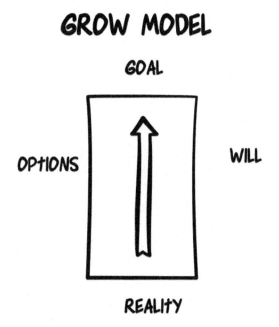

If you've done any work on goal-setting before, or attended a course that's looked at goal setting, then you may have heard of the acronym SMART. This is about goals being specific, meaningful, achievable, relevant, and time-bound. You will see that we do not include SMART on the GROW model, but of course, you can still bear in mind and use SMART alongside this if you wish. We suggest, for the purpose of getting familiar and comfortable with the GROW model, that you use the GROW in the sequence laid out below and just use the SMART words as a check list.

The goal – specific and purpose

There are two key elements to the goal:

The specifics about the goal. What is it in detail? Get as much specific information as possible about how big the goal is, when it should be achieved by, and any other details.

The purpose of the goal. This relates to why they want to achieve it. You really want to pull out the motivational drivers relating to pain, pleasure, intrinsic and extrinsic factors that we covered in the motivation chapter earlier. You don't want them to just state that achieving the goal will give them a pay rise, that's just part of it. Go deeper into the intrinsic drivers and understand what it will mean to them and their loved ones if they achieve this goal.

Examples of questions relating to the Specifics:

- What exactly do you want to achieve (short/long term)?
- By when do you want to achieve it?
- How much of this is within your own control?
- Is the goal positive, desirable, challenging, attainable?
- How will you measure it in terms of quality and quantity?
- Do you want to break down the overall goal into more manageable or realistic goals for this particular session?

Examples of questions relating to the Purpose (that will drive emotion and motivation):

- Why do you want to achieve it?

- How will it benefit you?
- What will it mean to you once you achieve it?
- What will the achievement say about you?
- How will that make you feel?
- How will that make anyone close to you feel knowing you feel that way?
- How will that make you feel ultimately knowing achieving the goal has done that?

Now you've understood from them what the specifics of the goal are and what the purpose is, note any key words or bullet points next to where it says **goal** on the paper.

Reality

In the next step, you should review the coachee's current strengths and weaknesses, as well as check and raise awareness of the situation and where they might be on the journey. What is the reality of where they are now? They could already be some way to achieving the goal, but may not have realised it.

Examples of questions:

- Where are you now with this goal?
- Why haven't you reached this goal already?
- What have you done so far to move towards this goal?
- What have you already learnt from that?
- Are there any constraints outside yourself which stop you moving towards this goal?
- How might you overcome them?
- What might you do to sabotage your own efforts to reach this goal?

Again, make some notes next to where it says **reality** on the paper.

Options

This is the fun part. Now it's time to brainstorm ways forward to find strategies, solutions, answers. Do not write anything off at this point and as a coach be conscious not to direct and tell if you can help it. Help the coachee to see what they could do to change the situation. What alternatives are there to that approach? Who could help? The coach's role is not primarily to provide answers. It is rather to stimulate creative ideas and possible actions that the coachee will more naturally buy into.

Examples of questions:

- What could you do to move towards this goal?
- What else could you do? And what else? (Keep repeating this!)
- If time was not a factor - what could you do?
- If resources were not a factor - what could you do?
- What would happen if you did nothing?
- Is there anybody whom you admire or respect who does this really well? What do they do which you could try?

Write all of the different options down the left hand side of the page where it says **options**. Try to fill the entire side of the page with all of the different ideas.

Will

Will covers two key elements:

What will they do and when?

What is their will power? How much do they want it?

It's now time to choose certain options and disregard others, test the commitment of the coachee to their goal, make concrete realistic plans to reach it and commit to action.

This involves identifying possible obstacles, making the next steps specific, agreeing timing, and identifying any support needed.

Examples of questions:

- Which of all the options will you choose? (Maybe several)
- When will you do this?
- When specifically (day, time) will you take the first step in your plan?
- How does this help you to achieve your goal?
- How will you know when you have reached your goal?
- Who else needs to know about your plan? How will you inform them?
- Who else needs to help and support you in your plan? How will you get that support?
- What obstacles do you expect to meet? How will you overcome them?

As the coachee chooses what they will do from the list of possible options, use arrows to point them to the right-hand side of the page. You're making a concrete list of what they will now do in order to achieve the goal. As you mark each option that they will do, try to include any relevant time frames.

Will power questions – you should ask all of these:

- How much do you really want to achieve this goal?
- What is your level of commitment to achieving this goal?
- How much do you want it on a scale of 1-10?

This is potentially the most critical questioning of all. Make sure you observe closely their commitment and ownership. If there is any sign of a lack of commitment, then refresh the 'purpose' element for the goal. Remind them of the intrinsic values behind them wanting to achieve it; their happiness, their pride, the fact their family will be proud. Hopefully this should encourage them to commit at a 10/10 level.

If they still fail to commit fully, then you have probably just wasted the past hour or so of your time as they are unlikely to achieve the goal! If they want it at a level of 6/10 and we think of it as a percentage, then they only want it 60%. That leaves 40% room for sabotage of the goal.

Do you think someone who allows 40% room for sabotage is likely to achieve it?

If you practice this exercise with different team members, and perhaps even friends and family, you will start to realise who is committed to achieving their goals and who isn't.

There will always be people who simply don't want to change, and will not take responsibility for themselves, and remember that the responsibility is theirs, not yours. Take confidence from those that appreciate your effort and for who this exercise will really help give them the direction they need to achieve.

See our example of a completed GROW model which should inspire you to start using this strategy with your team. As it's a visual model, you can keep copies on file to review during supervisions and appraisals, and they could also be anonymised for your CQC evidence folder too. We believe they are a great example for the well-led KLOE.

Using this model while practicing your coaching skills now completes the **What**, **How** and **Why** from the previous chapter. It helps to raise awareness and generate responsibility in the coachee and gives you a clear idea as to how you can facilitate their performance.

Studies have found that people are 42% more likely to achieve their goals if they are written down and so think of the difference this could make and the energy it could spark in your team if you complete this exercise with all of them.

You're now well on your way to becoming a great coach and hopefully empowering your staff to achieve awesome things for themselves too. But it's also important to look at how you can use coaching in negative circumstances too, and that's what we're going to look at in the next chapter.

GROW Model adapted from "Coaching For Performance" (third edition), by John Whitmore, 2002, Nicholas Brealey Publishing, London.

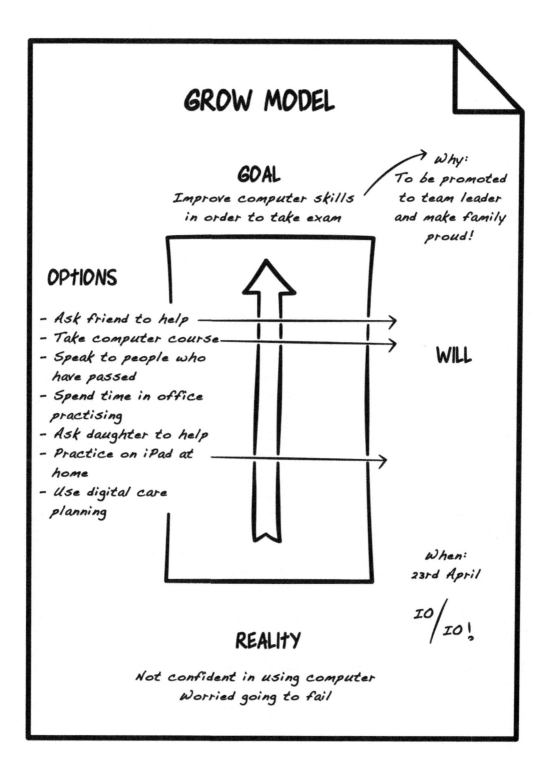

Giving feedback and having difficult conversations

Now you've become comfortable with the process of coaching it's time to use your new skills for a less enjoyable purpose, but one that will no doubt be necessary when you are a leader – giving feedback.

We have come across many leaders at all levels who struggle with having those difficult conversations or simply do not provide effective feedback that communicates what they really want to say.

Quite often, when giving a 'telling off' there can be emotions raised from either or both sides. We've looked, in earlier sections of this book, at what happens to performance when our own emotions 'run-a-mock' or we do not manage the emotions of who we are speaking with, and this is often the cause of feedback going badly. When emotions run high the outcome is not productive for either side.

This is where coaching can really make a difference. We know that it might seem strange to apply some of the coaching skills to giving feedback, but trust us, it really works. If you don't generally like having difficult conversations with staff or have ever avoided it altogether, then this will give you a framework to have a productive conversation and outcome.

A consideration before giving feedback is why you're giving it and what you want the outcome to be.

Reasons for giving feedback

Performance – You want the individual to learn and develop. This could be in an appraisal or supervision setting and is the most common reason for giving feedback.

Praise – Someone has done something that you think should be recognised and rewarded. It's interesting that this is reported by many as the least given form of feedback.

Emotional Rant – This may not be a legitimate form of feedback but it does happen a lot. Is there ever a benefit to an emotional rant? Well, you may gain some form of emotional release, but it inevitably creates guilt and pain too.

Consider what the person being ranted at will gain... They may be frightened and emotional enough to not make the mistake or performance error again. However, if you want the outcome to be learning and development then the emotional rant will contribute very little to that.

How feedback should be delivered

Although feedback can be communicated in different ways (such as in writing) the most common method is verbal feedback on performance, which could be given after someone has completed a task to a poor standard, or even something more serious, which requires disciplinary action.

Let's take a closer look at why this style of 'coached feedback' is often very powerful and the most appropriate way of having a feedback session. It also links very closely to the leadership styles and methods of communication which we looked at earlier.

It's worth pointing out that there will be occasions where this style of feedback is not appropriate and that may be because of time constraints or the severity of the situation. But, if the ideal outcome is for the person and for yourself to understand more about the situation, and for them to take in the feedback and be fully aware of what needs to happen as a result, then this is how you might best achieve that.

People who attend our Leadership Academies find that the feedback model we teach is not just useful for leaders who want to develop staff, it's also very effective for de-conflicting a potentially challenging scenario. It can be especially effective for leaders who are not comfortable with conflict or where there might be particularly challenging (or even aggressive) staff member.

Let's use an example:

Emma has had an argument with another colleague; Jane, in front of a resident and then stormed off, leaving Jane to do both of their tasks which caused her to run behind in her work. You decide to call Emma in to your office because you need to find out what happened.

The Feedback Model

The Feedback Model gives you steps to follow during the conversation, and they are:

1. Rapport
2. Explanation
3. Emotional impact
4. Needs to happen
5. Consequences and benefits
6. Close on commitment

An easy way to remember these is to think of the phrase: 'Randy Excited Elephants Need Careful Cuddling!' (or make up your own!) If you can remember that it can help you to write the first letter of each word in the corner of your notepad and the steps of the feedback model should come easily to you.

Rapport

You should aim to build rapport with Emma before launching into the conversation. It's important to try to make Emma feel as relaxed as possible as it will help manage the emotions of both parties and open a pathway for learning and trust.

This could be as simple as asking how she is and having open body language with her. If you have your arms crossed and look angry when she walks in then she will likely be defensive from the outset. Obviously, Emma will know why she has been called to you and might not relax completely, but if she sees that you are not going to start shouting then she should feel a bit calmer and more open to sharing.

Explanation

Now you will come to the main part of the conversation and will ask Emma for an explanation as to what happened. It's very important that you find out from her, rather than starting by telling her what you've been told.

When she is giving her explanation, try to ensure she is telling you the facts of the story, and not getting too emotional about it. You want the detail, but by keeping her to the facts it will ensure she doesn't go off on a tangent or begin getting upset or angry. Remember at this point that you are not giving any opinion, you are just gently prompting her by asking questions: "What happened" and "What happened next".

Emotional impact

Now that you've obtained the pure facts of the story from Emma, it's time to create some emotional impact so that she can see the results of her behaviour. To do that, start asking her questions that will allow her to see it for herself. You shouldn't tell her how she's made Jane feel. You should ask her: "How do you think that made Jane feel, when you left her to pick up your work?" and then "How do you think that makes me feel, to hear that you've shouted in front of a resident?"

Don't tell her, have the answers come from her. By recognising how her actions have impacted, she will feel the weight of what she's done much more than if you just told her. Ask her how she feels about this. She will probably now express that she feels bad and feels like she has let her colleague and you down.

Needs to happen

Again, using your questioning, coaching style, ask her what she thinks needs to happen now. It might surprise her to be asked what she thinks, instead of being told, but by answering and telling you: "I should apologise to Jane" and having that come from her means that she has taken responsibility for her actions.

Have you noticed that not once have we suggested you state anything to her? Ok, so in real life she may need some gentle prompting, but do your best to make everything you say a question, and that way you're avoiding conflict by letting everything come from her.

Consequences and benefits

Now that Emma has agreed what needs to happen next and any apologies or steps she needs to take to move forward, it's time to hit her with a small amount of pain, followed by a small amount of pleasure.

The pain is an emotional impact. Ask her what she thinks will happen if her behaviour doesn't improve. Let her acknowledge and tell you the consequences, perhaps she will be given a formal disciplinary or miss out on a promotion.

Then you want to highlight the benefits in order to give her some motivation to move forward. Ask her what could happen if she does take the steps to address her behaviour? She should acknowledge that it will create a better working atmosphere and she may be in with a chance of the promotion.

Close on commitment

Finally, before you let Emma go, confirm with her what she's now going to do and by when. By re-affirming her next steps you gain her commitment to move forward.

By asking questions throughout, it puts you in control of the conversation and helps you to lead Emma to a successful outcome, without putting pressure on you to 'tell her off'.

tHE FEEDBACK MODEL

R	RAPPORt

E	EXPLANAtION

E	EMOtIONAL IMPACt

N	NEEDS tO BE DONE

C	CONSEQUENCES / BENEFItS

C	CLOSE ON COMMItMENt

Challenges

Not every feedback session will be smooth sailing, so we wanted to address a few of the typical challenges people face when using the Feedback Model.

Potential Challenge 1 – Understanding fact from fiction

You've asked Emma to explain what happened, but what if her story is different from Jane? It is important for the explanation to come from Emma initially, as you then get to understand her 'map of the world' - and if she genuinely thinks that's what happened, it's relevant to moving forward as you may have to create doubt about her belief and prove to her exactly what happened.

This may have to come in the form of using methods such as showing video evidence, but it could be as simple as gently challenging the facts.

If you need to do this be sure not to begin any sentence with: "In my opinion..." Your opinion may not be a fact and will not change Emma's understanding of what happened or her development unless you can keep her to the facts.

Potential challenge 2 – I don't know

It can be very frustrating to ask questions and be met with the answer: "I don't know" so the best way to handle this is to gently prompt again: "But what if you did know?"

Do your best to tease out the answer from them, because it means their awareness is raised and you are generating responsibility

Potential challenge 3 – No engagement

Again, this is tricky and frustrating but if someone will not engage at all in your questioning then either take a break for them to cool off or you may have to resort to the 'tell' style, but still using the framework. In each section attempt to extract the information from them if you can. The most important part is 'close on commitment' and ensure they tell you their action points. If they fail to do this then our suggestion would be to put it in writing to them and have them sign it, but at this stage you may be forced to take further disciplinary action.

We hope that going forward you become more and more comfortable using the Feedback Model and consider using it for positive feedback too.

Even if you've been comfortable giving feedback to people in the past, by using this model it really does help to de-escalate any situations that could potentially get heated and allow for the person you're giving feedback to see it as a constructive conversation, with you firmly in control.

Developing confidence

We will begin with a definition of confidence and we like this definition as it expresses a level of humility:

Confidence means feeling sure of yourself and your abilities — not in an arrogant way, but in a realistic, secure way. Confidence isn't about feeling superior to others. It's a quiet inner knowledge that you're capable. Confident people feel secure, rather than insecure.

Developing confidence in care staff is a regular challenge we are tasked with, and particularly, we see a lack of confidence in newly promoted leaders. This can impact again and again as people jump up through promotions so if you are a new team leader reading this and feel under-confident, just know that your boss will have probably had the same feelings when they started in their new role. This chapter is for anyone who wants to build confidence in themselves or others, or perhaps both.

To understand why we might lack confidence it helps to know what factors make us less confident when doing certain things or striving for specific goals. The Performance Spiral from the first section of the book illustrates the relationship between mindset, emotions and behaviour and confidence sits within the mindset part of the spiral.

Whilst it's part of mindset, being under-confident then has an impact on emotions and attitude and so on around the spiral. Go and refresh yourself on the graphics from that chapter if you need to. Remember that the key components we shared within the mindset domain were self-image, beliefs and vision, all can be impacted on by what we are saying in our heads - our self-talk. The crux to developing confidence is to know what factors are undermining it and how to apply an intervention.

It's also important to know that if you are helping someone to develop their confidence it is no use saying: "Come on, just be confident", as that gives only your opinion and doesn't consider the thoughts of the petrified team leader, who is moments from giving their first public speech. How many times have you been told: "Just be confident" and it didn't shift your confidence one bit?!

Let's explore the components and a strategy for developing confidence by working through and smashing any hurdles the various components may throw up. This can be used in a wide range of scenarios and it's especially good for developing yourself, members of staff and even your friends and family.

Firstly, we must establish what it is that creates the confidence issue and that could be inside or outside of work. We have come across a range of scenarios that impact on the confidence of people, so think about what yours could be. It's not always obvious. Sometimes someone who appears super confident may not be in certain scenarios. The extroverted ringleader of a small clique is often someone who is less confident than the impression they try and give!

If you or someone else lacks confidence in a certain scenario then a few typical things that will be happening:

- The internal communication and self-talk will be negative, such as: "I'm going to be useless" or "there is no way I can do that."
- Belief in the ability to succeed will be limiting and not empowering. We are going to look at this in more detail shortly. This will be compounded by the negative self-talk.
- Emotions will start to influence both an ability to think logically, control behaviour and even bodily functions. Shaking and flushed faces are common.

The strategy for developing confidence

The intervention to develop confidence has therefore got to address all three areas above otherwise there will still be a barrier standing in the way and regardless of what you do you will never be fully confident.

The areas are; self-talk, belief and emotional control or EQ. We're not going to tackle emotional control in this chapter as we've already covered it at length and recommend going back to the EQ section and particularly the State Management exercise. In this section we are going to look specifically at overcoming negative self-talk and limiting beliefs.

tHE SELF CONCEPt MODEL

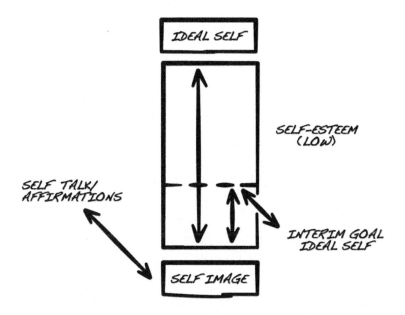

Addressing Self-Image

A common cause for negative internal communication is because of self-image, which is how we see ourselves or can sometimes be referred to as 'what we see when we look in the mirror.' This can be in general or specific to a scenario.

As well as self-image, we also have an 'ideal self' which is what we would ideally like to see, or how we would like to perform in a scenario.

If our self-image is negative, and we see ourselves as inadequate (bear in mind this can be influenced by other people) and our self-image is far away from our ideal self, then this can drive down self-esteem and confidence and in turn, make us feel even more negative about ourselves.

Note that this is now very much about feelings and sits within the 'emotions' part of the performance spiral.

If you're working with someone to improve their confidence then first establish how to improve their self-image.

The intervention to develop self-image and self-esteem is:

Self-talk

Establish what they're saying in their head that is driving a low self-image. The words are likely to be negative. Help them to create one or two affirmations that will define their desired emotion for when they have to perform in a scenario. As we've discussed previously with affirmations, the key is make the words about what they want to do and not what they don't want to do.

For example, if a member of staff has a low self-image around having to deal with someone from the local authority and says: "I'll be rubbish" or "I will mess things up" then they should have affirmation words such as 'strong' or 'calm' that will help them create the right self-image before the meeting.

Set interim goals

Reduce the gap between self-image and ideal self by setting achievable short-term goals that can be reached quickly en route to the overall ideal self. Rewards should be built in along the way to the overall goal. By doing this it closes the gap between ideal self and self-image and providing the successes and improvement are celebrated along the way then self-esteem should improve.

The best example of this is with weight loss clubs. If someone wants to lose two stone then it can seem impossible because the ideal self is so far away. Most weight loss clubs build in smaller achievable goals along the way, such as a half stone milestone to be celebrated, and this can help build a sense of achievement and boost self-esteem along the way.

How can you replicate this with someone on your own team who may have an ideal self, but is struggling with negative self-talk and low self-image? What affirmations could they create? What interim goals could they set? These are relatively simple, yet powerful ways of building self-confidence.

Now let's look at belief which can have a real impact on low self-confidence.

Challenging Limiting Beliefs

An empowering belief is a belief that we can do something, whilst a limiting belief is a belief that we can't do something.

Earlier in the book we shared that limiting beliefs are inbuilt within us to protect us from doing something that can cause us harm, but the problem is we can go overboard with them, and they can stop us achieving great things.

To create an empowering belief, we simply must override the limiting belief with a new powerful belief that we can succeed. It's not always simple though, it depends on how fixed and strong the limiting belief is.

In order to override the limiting belief, we need to challenge where the belief came from and try to discredit the things which are holding us back. This could be because someone has once told us we couldn't do something, or because we've had a bad experience in the past. Whatever it is, it's about reframing that belief so it goes from: "I can't" to "Maybe I could" to "I can."

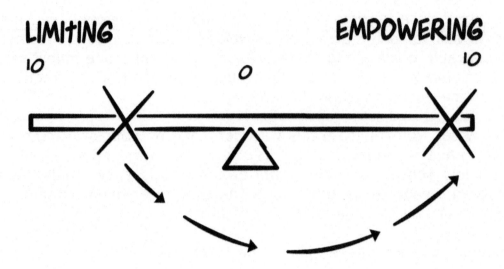

Exercise

If someone on your team has a limiting belief that they can't do something, and this could be technical or something like the previous example of having to deal with the local authority, then remember your coaching skills. It's important not to take ownership by 'telling' but focus on asking questions to open their mind:

- What is the limiting belief you have about a certain scenario? What is it you believe you can't do?
- Where did the belief come? Where is the evidence that you can't do it?

Here you need to establish exactly what is propping up this belief and what the evidence and facts are. As they begin to tell you why they can't do something you should start to create doubt by challenging the evidence. Some of it will be easy to squash as they realise they may not have many real reasons as to why they can't do it. Some may be because someone has told them they can't do something or because they've tried and failed before.

For example: "A previous manager told me I would never pass my NVQ" or: "I've never done anything like that before."

You want to understand why the previous manager would have said that and create doubt by saying: "How can they say you wouldn't pass?" and "What do they know? That's just their opinion, not fact." As you start to create doubt about the limiting belief you should introduce questions that help to create an empowering belief such as: "Didn't you pass the care certificate?" and "Have you passed other exams in the past? So why not this one!" You will know when you have created a shift and it can be a really uplifting moment when it happens. Suddenly there is hope.

Once the doubt has been created and you are at the possibility stage you have to continue and build this through to an empowering belief.

To build the empowering belief move through a goal setting activity exploring options to help and make it happen. Ask questions such as: "If you spoke with Hayley who passed her NVQ do you think that would help?" and "Could you find some time to study and I can test you once a week? Do you think that would help?"

Continue to build the empowering belief until you can ask them: "If you do all of this then now do you think you can achieve it?" They should now have smashed that limiting belief and overridden it with an empowering one. Picture the graphic on the previous page as you progress, or even a seesaw tipping from one way to the other.

Whilst working on confidence with someone in your team, there are some things to be cautious of:

Remember when creating any affirmations that they should be positive. "Don't get nervous" is a negative affirmation! Never have an affirmation that says what you shouldn't do – it should always say what you should do, such as: "Be calm."

It can be useful to establish scores whenever coaching. When they say they can't do something, ask how much they feel that out of 10. You'll know if it's a really strong limiting belief (if they say 10/10 they can't do it) and as you coach them into overcoming it you can ask for ratings again as you move the marker to zero and then up into an empowering belief of: "10/10 I can do it!"

Be sure to create doubt by questioning. We can't emphasise this enough. If they express something that is a belief, you can't say: "Don't be ridiculous!" you need to prove to them otherwise. If they say they are nervous then you should ask questions such as: Have you ever been nervous before but got through it? What did you do?"

When you reach the tipping point of the belief; when it starts to become an empowered belief, it may be time to start a goal setting exercise such as the Grow Model to help build on it.

After the scenario, exam or whatever it may be has happened review everything with them, with a focus on the key strengths. Give praise and reinforce the confidence that has been built. On any aspects that could have gone better simply review them and create action to address them so that the belief will be even more empowered for next time.

Confidence cannot be built overnight. You will have people on your team who will be underconfident in things and from the outside you may not be able to understand why. But by working through these exercises and overcoming any limiting beliefs they may have you help to build them up and this will have an impact on their motivation, self-leadership and overall wellbeing.

To be able to develop confidence in the people around you is one of the most powerful tools you can have as a leader, so practice, practice practice! We promise it will be worth it and you will see remarkable achievements from your team, but don't be afraid to try this with underconfident teenagers and see what they too can achieve with your support.

Leading others – summary

It wouldn't be possible to learn all of this section in one go and suddenly become a fantastic leader of others. It all takes time, and as we've said, that's why coaching is one of the least used leadership styles, not just in care but across all industries.

If you can find the time to start practicing these techniques and exercises, starting with people you feel comfortable with, then before long you'll start to see the difference in the people around you. Their confidence will grow, the team will become more motivated and as a leader you will feel more comfortable in your own abilities to lead.

Don't just focus on your team. We see people get great results from using the exercises from this section with their kids, teenagers, partners, scout clubs and knitting societies!

Come back and refresh yourself when you need to. If things don't go to plan then review and coach yourself to get better. You will get there. It takes work but it's worth it.

Part 3

Leading The Culture

Developing The Culture

The true test for any leader, is to take the culture of the home or company and develop it into a truly positive workplace. Sometimes it can seem like an impossible challenge, especially with every other responsibility you have, but if you can crack it then you will improve every aspect of the business; recruitment, retention, care quality, wellbeing and everything in between.

Think about the best place you ever worked... is there somewhere that stands out? Think about what made that place special. Was it the people? Your boss? The job itself? How much did the company culture factor into what you loved about it? It was probably a key factor.

What is culture?

Culture is personality or the vibe of the workplace. It defines the environment in which people work. It's the feel of the place, it's how you do things, it's the character. It's quite often built on the company values or mission statement and it can be led by the owner, manager or the people.

Culture can be positive or negative and culture can change, either naturally or with some effort. We like to think that the culture drives the behaviours of the people that work there and so it's arguably the most important part of your leadership - to get the culture right.

> **Side note:** If you are not the owner or manager of a care company then don't skip this chapter, as you can still have an impact on the culture of your immediate team. If you are part of a bigger group, with a marketing department who is defining the culture from above, then again you can still have an impact. This chapter is relevant whether you are an owner, a manager or a team leader, in a large organisation or a single care home.

Your own culture

How would you describe your current culture? Overall, is it positive or negative? Would you say it is a learning culture; where people are happy to teach and mentor each other? Is there a 'cliquey' culture where new people struggle to fit in with well-established teams? Is there more of a flat culture which is when people feel they can talk to management and share any thoughts, ideas or concerns? Is there a results-oriented culture and everyone is striving for the next award or improved CQC rating?

It's important to think about where you are now and what you'd like to change. There may be a dramatic change needed, or it may be more subtle. But one thing's for sure – in order to drive change into a company culture you're going to have to get people on board.

Assessing your culture

To get people thinking about the culture and raise your awareness of what the team are perceiving, we like a little game called Culture Mad Libs. If you've never played Mad Libs before, it's a game where you fill in blank spaces in a story to create funny, nonsensical stories. However, for Culture Mad Libs, you're going to get a real sense of what words your team use to describe the culture.

Use the template provided or download it from the website to print: **www.careleadershandbook.co.uk**

We recommend you give it a go yourself first and just fill it in with the words you would use now, not in an ideal world. Then give printed copies of the worksheet to the team and have them fill it in and return to you, and make sure they can do this anonymously.

Before doing that, it would be good to let the team know why you are having them complete this crazy exercise in the first place. Mention it at a staff meeting and just say you're really interested to know more from their perspective how they feel about the culture and that the little Mad Libs game is just a starting point to gain some insight.

CULTURE MADLIBS

I feel .... to be working at ....
      [emotion]   [company]

This morning I walked into the .... and the first thing I saw was
                                [room or space]

.... which is very typical here because
[something you might see]

....
          [why]

My manager says people who do well here are .... , ... and
                                [adjective]   [adjective]

....
  [adjective]

Our staff meetings are often .... and ....
                            [describe what the meetings are like]

.... often happens.
[describe what happens]

If I stay here it will be because .... And if I go it would be because
                       [best thing about working for the company]

.... The first rule of working here is ....
[why people leave]   [the thing that's important]

but if you want to really succeed here you need to remember

....
[unwritten rule that everyone abides by]

When you've got the worksheets back it's time to review – you may want to do this with a large coffee or even a glass of wine! Look for common words and themes running through the worksheets. Make notes of repeating words and reflect what's being perceived by the team in comparison to your own perception.

Set aside some time to thank the team for their contribution and feed back to them what you've learned from the exercise and what you plan to do going forward.

Now it's time for the next phase in your journey to develop the culture.

Bringing company values to life

Your company values are going to be a key factor in your new or improved company culture. But what do your company values represent right now? Are they just words on the website or a wall of head office? If you stopped someone from your team in the corridor and asked them what the company values are, would they be able to tell you?

If you don't know the answer to this then go and try it right now! Put the book down and go and ask someone what your company values are. That's test number one. If they know what they are then test number two is to ask them what the values mean. This may catch them out. You might find they can't articulate what it actually means to embody those values within the company.

This is what we are going to change.

More than words on a page

We are presuming you do have a set of company values, but if you don't then that's fantastic and you can still go through this whole process to create your values from scratch.

At this point, it's worth us mentioning that people often stop us and say: "our company values are dictated by head office so there's nothing we can do to change them" and this is a fair point. But, while you may not be able to change the words, there are things you can do to develop them into more than just words.

So, if your values, and therefore an element of your culture is being dictated from the top, what can you do to develop them?

Think about Harry Potter. You may not be a fan, but we are sure you're aware that at Hogwarts (the school for witchcraft and wizardry) there were four houses; Griffindor, Ravenclaw, Hufflepuff and Slytherin. Now, the school had its own mission statement that was about Hogwarts being a nourishing environment and encouraging pupils to perform at the best of their abilities. But, the individual houses, whilst falling under the overall mission statement, also had their own values. Griffindor was about courage and chivalry, Hufflepuff was about patience and loyalty... and so on.

Do you see that you can have company values, but the houses within the company can still have quite different personalities or character and still sit under the over-arching values?

Hopefully this is useful if you are part of a larger group and it might be useful to think about the other homes in your region and how you would describe their personality or culture in comparison to your own.

The problem with care company values

The biggest problem we find with care company values, is that they're often the same as each other. In fact, lots of company values across many industries are often the same, but care in particular often features values such as: Caring, Dignity, Respect, Compassion, Integrity, Understanding.

Did you smile reading those? Was one of your company values listed? We often ask audiences to put their hand up if they have a value of 'respect' and many hands will go up.

The problem with having the same values as every other care company is that the meaning of those values can quite often be lost, and there's nothing to differentiate between one company to another.

So, if you use your company values as they currently stand to try to create movement in your culture, then right now they may just fall on deaf ears, because they don't mean anything to the staff. Imagine if we said to you: "Your values are X, Y and Z". Not many people would appreciate having values dictated to them if they didn't necessarily agree with those values or buy-in to them.

In order to create culture change, you need to develop the values into more than just words. You need to develop them into entire culture statements that are created, owned, lived and breathed by the staff. **Culture Statements** is your next project.

How to develop culture statements

In order to create culture statements with your team you need to gather them together for a workshop. We realise this is not always easy in a busy care environment so think about how you can do this without leaving people out.

If you're a manager of an entire home you might want to take groups, or if you are a team leader you might do this with just your immediate team.

If they've already done the Mad Libs exercise then they will have already given some thought to the culture of the company, so explain that this is the next step and that you'd like to figure out, with them, how you can bring the company values to life, and use them to develop a positive workplace culture.

How to run a culture statements workshop

You'll need coloured pens and paper, but you might also want post-it notes and a white board or flip chart.

Set the scene with the team and explain this is an open workshop and that you'd like everyone to contribute.

Start by writing the company values on different pieces of paper. If you've got flipchart paper you can pin them up on different walls of the room.

Split people into groups, give them pens and have them each take a piece of paper with one of the values on it and ask them to brainstorm around the word. For example, 'respect'. What does respect mean to them in your home? What would they like it to mean? Be clear this is about them, rather than what it would mean for the clients.

Have them debate it first, and then scribble down as many statements as they can think of as to what respect means, and also what they would like it to mean in the home.

Sophie says: *"I've taught this workshop to groups of managers before and I've found some struggle to grasp the concept of this exercise. I've had managers say that their value of 'respect' can only ever mean respect for clients. But remember this exercise is not about clients and you'll find that your team might be able to come up with many different definitions of respect and get really creative in this workshop."*

Give them 10 minutes and then rotate the groups so that each group gets to scribble their own ideas on each piece of paper. Have them circle any previous scribblings that they like, and that way it will highlight the most popular statements on each piece of paper.

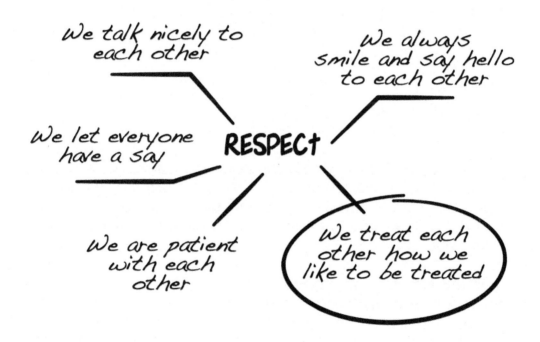

Once every group has written on every value then it's time to review.

Have someone from each group read out the value and the statements. Is there a clear winner? If not let the group debate it but make sure you keep track of the time and take a vote if needed. Ideally, you'll end up with one statement for each of the values.

So now you have a set of values and a set of statements that define more clearly what the values mean. These have been created and agreed by the team as a set of statements they would like everyone to embody in the home. Thank everyone for their contributions and let them know this is just the beginning! Now the fun starts.

What to do with your culture statements

Now you have the statements created, it would be good to make a bit of a fuss about them. No doubt, you will have people on the team who may have rolled their eyes at the workshop and wondered what the point of it was. We've all worked for companies where they've started a project that just seems to fade into distant memory within a few weeks.

Your mission is to now drive these statements forward into the behaviours of the people working in the home and the best way to start that is with visual reinforcement.

Put up a notice board, create posters and make sure the new culture statements are prominently displayed around the home. If you send out a staff newsletter or bulletin, make sure they are in there and don't forget all of this can be recorded for your evidence folder for CQC.

Even if you already had a good working culture, don't be afraid to communicate the purpose of the workshop and the culture statements to relatives and clients themselves – the impact of driving an improved culture will reach to them too, and the more people who understand what your culture is all about, the quicker it will become embedded.

Start a recognition campaign. Perhaps people could nominate each other for things that they have done that demonstrate the new culture statements. Once a month you could have a 'Culture Club' winner and make sure their story is shared on your notice board, in any newsletters and across social media. We saw a care company who had theirs in a frame at reception so that any visitor could read about the member of staff who had brought the values to life in their work that month.

By doing this, the culture statements will remain fresh in the team's minds while they go about their day to day activities. You will know they are truly embedded when the team begin to self-police the statements and call each other out if they feel someone is not living by the statements they helped create. This is really driving a self-leadership culture; where everyone takes responsibility for the culture they are helping to create and if you see this happening in your home then you know the shift is happening.

Make your culture statements go further

Now that the statements are becoming a natural guidance for every day life in the home, it's time to think about how you can use them on a wider scale. If the statements are really being lived and breathed within the home and the staff are taking ownership of them, then you want to ensure that anyone else coming into the home is aware of, and wants to embody these values. Here are some tips on how to do this:

Social Media

Lots of people struggle to find content to put in their social media posts but the culture statements help to give you lots of content ideas. You can share who has won the Culture Club for the month which shows that you recognise and reward staff for their hard work.

You could post photos of everyone in the culture statement workshops (with their permission of course) and this demonstrates that you are gaining the insight from staff and involving them in what the culture of the company should be.

You can also regularly post reminders about the culture statements within the home and how they guide the staff and are put into practice.

Think about who will see these posts. People who are looking for a job may look through your social media before applying and will see a culture where staff are involved in its' development. Any potential staff who want this kind of empowerment will know straight away that your home is the right environment for them. They've already been shown your culture statements and how people behave within the home. This can really help to attract the right type of staff.

Potential clients or their relatives may also have a nosy through your social media before making an appointment to visit, and they will get a good feel for the place through what you post. The culture of the staff within the home will have a huge impact on the residents so this could be a real positive for any potential client. Bear in mind they will walk through those doors expecting to feel that culture, so make sure those notice boards, monthly "culture club" winners and the staff behaviour reflects what you're posting on social media!

Existing staff should be proud to work there and hopefully they too follow the company on social media. They should be encouraged to share the culture-related posts and as they do we are sure you will find more and more new staff applications come from friends and relatives of your existing team.

Your website

We list your website separately to social media as the website is often the more formal, clinical overview of the company. If you have a blog then it would be worth having one on the process of developing the culture statements. If not, you could have something on the 'About Us' page which describes them. Make it clear that any mission statement or values are aimed at the clients, but that the culture statements are there for the staff.

Job descriptions

When was the last time you refreshed your job post adverts or job descriptions? The culture statements give you an opportunity to make yours stand out from any competition. Instead of the boring list of skillset requirements you can now describe the sort of people that will fit in with the culture.

By doing this you will generate more of an emotional connection with any applicants – they will remember what they've read and know they are the right fit.

At interview

Now you can review your interview questions and use the culture statements to form some scenario-based interview questions. By asking the interviewee how they would behave in certain scenarios means you can test if they will likely fit into the culture that you're all working so hard to develop.

Hopefully, if people are doing their research by looking at your social media and have properly read the job description then they will naturally be a better fit for your company, and this will come across in their answers.

The welcome letter

Later we will share the importance of a welcome letter and the culture statements are something you can work into that too. Perhaps you'll have had some reminder cards made with the statements on them and you can include those in the letter or even written into the handbook.

However you choose get the message across, it's important to let the new starter know how important these statements are, and how they're owned by the staff.

Induction

By incorporating the culture statements into the induction process, it will help the new member of staff to fit in and quickly become adjusted to the way of life in the company. They will probably already have a good feel for the culture through the recruitment process, but make sure the statements and any visual reinforcement is explained to them so that they know it's not just words on a wall and will factor into a successful induction.

Recognition

Ensure that any Culture Club winners don't just get praise within the company, send a letter to their home with a card or handwritten note explaining what they did to win and how much it means that they're living the culture. Their family may be curious to hear more and this is helping to share the message that you are a company that values staff.

Family don't always realise what goes into care and may also be subject to the more negative stories about the job, so this is a great way to include them in your positive culture initiative and keep them informed.

Appraisals and supervisions

One to one time with staff members is a great time to refresh and reinforce the culture statements. If you can work them into the appraisal process then they won't be forgotten and will continue to drive the culture forward in the company.

Culture ambassadors

A great way of giving extra responsibility to people in the company is to put together a small group of culture ambassadors – the people who can really influence and drive the culture change. Let them come up with new ideas on how to drive the culture, let them get creative.

Make sure that new people get to spend time with them so that their energy rubs off. Ensure that they have good lines of open communication with management so that they can report any issues or resistance so that it can be dealt with quickly.

So there you have it! Potentially a mammoth task to really drive culture change in your company, but one that can have so many benefits and really make a difference to the quality of the staff you attract and retain. You may find that once you're on this journey there will be people who are not willing to get on board; and where possible we advise having quite a mercenary approach to those who won't adapt to change. Bad apples can have a very negative impact on a team and quickly drive a negative culture that could ruin any progress you are making.

Your culture ambassadors should be able to spot and report this to you, and just be aware that some people like to complain and be stuck in a negative environment. Who knows why! It's not a failure on your part if you can't flip them, perhaps it is time to support them to find gainful employment elsewhere!

Leaders who truly invest in developing their culture reap the benefits. When you see staff begin to self-police and reinforce the culture then you'll know you've cracked it. When you have staff who are driving forward the agreed culture, then you'll find it easier to do the job of leading. You'll be able to delegate more, staff will sort out small issues between themselves without relying on you and you will have an overriding culture of self-leadership within the team. Wouldn't that be the dream?

Team cohesion

A key element to drive positive workplace culture can be team cohesion.

Rob says: *"Team Cohesion is a state of behaviour, values, emotion and mindset and relates directly to the stickability and inter-dependent support that a team has working together for a common purpose."*

Recognise the words in this description and reflect back to some of the earlier sections of the book which looked at the performance spiral, goal setting, developing the values and culture. All of these will impact on team cohesion and it's likely that if you've been working your way through the book with your team then you will already be noticing a developing relationship between them.

Have you ever been in a team that just 'had it'? That spirit, energy and togetherness, regardless of the various personality types within the team? If you have, then wonderful things will have happened. You probably hit targets, got great feedback from the people you were supporting, plenty of referrals from them and they will have actively promoted you. The people within that team would also have spoken highly about the team and had a sense of pride being part of it. That says it all really, if you have a high level of team cohesion then your team will get on, support each other and work with a positive attitude that will impact on referrals and client satisfaction.

Consider how important referrals and client satisfaction is to your business? These things will impact on every aspect of your care company including care quality, CQC reports and even company profits.

Personality impacts on team cohesion

When it comes to personality it's interesting that you can have opposite personality types and yet still get on. Perhaps your best friend and you are like this? Or your sibling? What you more likely have in common are your values-based behaviours.

Have you ever heard someone say: "Our personalities clashed"? Yet you most likely have friends with all different personalities and get on fine with each of them. The clash was more likely between values-based behaviours than personality.

When there is good team cohesion, providing there is a high level of social awareness and social management then we tend to behave appropriately and by sharing what our likes, dislikes and preferences of communication and support are it will help massively with how a team function - especially in challenging scenarios. Different personalities do not mean that a team can't have good team cohesion.

Managing personality types

There are some considerations when leading and managing different personality types. Here we will just focus on two general types - introverts and extroverts. Even if you or they have not taken a personality test you can have a good idea if someone is introverted or extroverted based on their behaviour and the way they communicate.

An extrovert tends to be outgoing and outspoken and will enjoy being around people. An introvert tends to be more self-contained and reserved.

We will all have degrees of both in us and in some cases those degrees could be extreme. For example, you could be an over the top extrovert - the life and soul of the party.

It is important to understand that regardless of personality, if we are in high self-image and emotionally balanced, we will tend to behave and communicate appropriately, regardless of personality type. It's when we are highly emotional or have low self-image that we tend to drift towards the negative traits of our personality, and that can cause issues within teams.

Referring back to the Performance Spiral you will know that it's important to manage emotions in order to control behaviour so this is how to support the different personality types when their emotional Richter scale is starting to rise:

Introverts in a low self-image and stressed state:

- Body language will be withdrawn and closed down.
- Language will be passive and quiet.
- Negotiation and discussion will be weak. They may surrender to any challenge in order to remove themselves from the situation. They will lose, the other person wins.
- Bear in mind that introverts may still reach a tipping point and get hostile.

With introverts you need to give them space and time to recharge if they are feeling under pressure. When they're ready you should help them to feel heard by promoting their ideas and encouraging them to find their voice.

Extroverts in a low self-image and stressed state:

- Body language will be large and aggressive, and they will try and dominate by putting people down to make their self-image feel better (This doesn't work but can be a common trait).
- Language will be inappropriate and threatening.
- Negotiation will be either: win for them and lose for you or lose/lose for both as there is no way they will want you to win - even if they lose as well.

Extroverts need to be pacified and made to feel comfortable. You may want to put them down if they are being too loud but putting them down reduces their self-image further, increases stress and the scenario could potentially get worse. This is the time to reason, control their emotions and then negotiate in a logical way.

Now let's move on from this brief look at personality types and look at developing team cohesion based on elements we've covered earlier.

Developing team cohesion

Team cohesion will directly reflect the culture and values of your team and so using the development strategies discussed earlier in the book will help massively. However, let's take a look at some other key aspects of measuring and developing it and the evidence that suggests this is a critical factor in being a successful high performing team.

TEAM COHESION

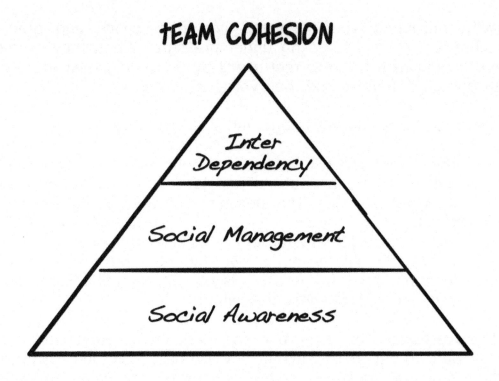

Inter Dependency

Social Management

Social Awareness

We call this triangle a taxonomy which means the base element influences the next tier up and then that tier influences the top tier. We have already discussed the base and middle tier which are **social awareness** and **social management** in the first section of this book, when we took a deep dive into Emotional Intelligence. Do you remember the example of a team of 6 having 36 points of contact? If not, go back and refresh yourself. The final and top tier is a measure of **interdependency**.

Interdependency is when every member of a team will support, step in to help and totally back each other up when they are on the job. It's not to say everyone is best friends or they won't have a row on occasion, it's just that they 100% trust and support each other. Interdependency could be impacted if there are people in the team who are less skilled so can't support in that sense, however willingness and moral support are often more important.

If you have had chance to review the elements of social awareness and social management from the earlier chapter, you should now have a good picture of what makes up some key elements of team cohesion. It's now time to measure these and this can be done with just some simple reflections on what the ideal would look like in each element and bench mark your own team against this.

Also, understand that this is your perception and other members of the team may have different opinions which will be true to them. Referring to the Spiral, if they think and believe it, it will generate an emotion and subsequent action, and therefore it's critical for a leader to know what the team think and feels even though it maybe a mile away from your own opinion. Just understanding this increases Social Awareness!

Combined, the quality of each tier will go a long way in predicting the cohesion of a team so here is what you can do as an exercise.

Measuring Team Cohesion:

- Do this on your own initially to give yourself a good reflection of the team. Then consider bringing the team into it and do this as a group activity. Explain the purpose and what you want to achieve.
- Explain each element starting with Social Awareness, then Social Management and finally Interdependency and ask them to rate what they think the team scores, 1 being poor and 10 being ideal, on the scale. Ensure you get everybody's individual perceived score and then take an average of each area.
- Once you have the scores engage the team in what is positive and negative about the actions, behaviours and attitudes of the team.

- Then using the same strategy as you would on a wheel and GROW model create an action plan to go forward. Ensure you build in a future action review, as with all goal setting.
- These activities will need consistent review, resetting and driving. It's essential behaviours become habit and this in turn creates fantastic team cohesion and a great culture.

Wheel of performance – for teams

Remember the wheel of performance that we covered earlier? We're now going to look at how you can take that exercise and expand it into a full team workshop that's ideal for understanding the team's perceptions of the company. This is a different type of workshop to the culture statements one, because that was about deciding and developing the culture, whereas this is about spotting collective development areas within the team. This workshop will still impact the culture if you can find areas to be improved and it shows that you are taking steps to facilitate performance with the team.

Hopefully you've now got the hang of completing the wheel with individuals so it's a great time to move onto the whole team. Now depending on your set up this might be something you can do with your entire staff at once, or it might be easier to break it down into different teams or areas. So, for example if you run a care home with a kitchen department, admin department and different care teams you may wish to conduct the exercise with each different department. We do appreciate it's not always easy to gather the entire staff team together at once!

Let's say you've taken the care team and you're in a lounge for a staff meeting. Now instead of taking each spoke of the wheel as the role, you want to be looking at the **qualities** that make up the home or department. Let's say we are looking at the whole home. The spokes of the wheel might be things like professionalism, teamwork, humour, processes, leadership. Let the group choose and make sure you have a large piece of paper or flipchart to mark the wheel out on.

WHEEL OF PERFORMANCE

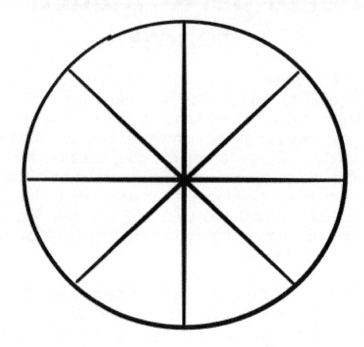

Once you've chosen what the eight (or less if time is pushed) spokes are start exactly as you would with an individual. Take the first spoke and ask them to describe what a ten out of ten would be for 'teamwork' as an example. Make sure everyone has a fair chance to speak and ensure people don't jump ahead and start rating too soon. Once everyone is in agreement (and feel free to a make a note of these descriptions) then ask them to consider where they would rate the home right now. Start at 10 and work your way down to zero asking for a quick show of hands until you can determine an average score for the group. Then note it, fill in the spoke and move onto the next one.

Remember the steps, just like in the individual performance wheels:

1. Define the spokes of the wheel
2. Describe what a 10/10 would look like
3. Rate and score the company/team now
4. Challenge the score and adjust if needed

Note that if there is a big difference in opinion you may need to listen and mediate, but resist telling anyone that they are wrong and watch out for others who may state that people's individual opinions are wrong. Make sure you challenge effectively, using open questions if necessary.

As a group exercise this can be a real eye-opener for a manager or team leader. There may be a real disconnect in how the team perceive the home and it's a really powerful way of better understanding where the home or company can focus on improvement.

If you're not a manager then you may still want to do this exercise with your immediate team so that you can feed back to senior management the results. There's nothing like seeing numbers on a page to inspire people to take action!

Sophie says: *"Depending on your relationship with the team you may find they are resistant to share their true feelings for fear of repercussions. If the session is contracted properly then this shouldn't be a problem but bear in mind you may get a truer result by having another member of your senior team host the exercise"*

Now the exercise is complete it's important to let the team know what you're going to do with the information and when you will follow up with them on it. There may be some simple improvements, or you may need a bigger action plan depending on that that wheel looks like, but now you are armed with information that can lead to change.

Keep records of all of this for your evidence folder for CQC. Perhaps take a few photos during the meeting and of the team wheel that you can include along with a brief write up as to why you did this exercise, what the key points raised were and what your action plan will be moving forward.

Staff induction

You may wonder why we've put a chapter on staff induction in this book as it's more of a process than a leadership skill. However, we find induction is often not given enough thought in a care company, but when done right it can really have a positive impact on new members of the team, help build a positive working culture and reduce staff turnover.

Why good induction is so important

At the time of printing, staff turnover in care is said to be 30.7%. Most companies tell us that they lose the majority of staff within the first three months, maybe even the first few weeks after they start.

In fact, 60% of staff who leave in the first year at a company state poor induction as a major factor in their decision.

Sometimes it just doesn't work out with a new hire but think about how many you could potentially save by having a really solid induction process in place. Studies have found that an effective induction process can cut staff turnover within the first year by up to 50%. How much do you think that would save you in terms of recruitment costs, advertising, time, training and the necessary background checks?

The maths

Let's say you have 100 people working in your home and your staff turnover sits around about the average; 30%. So, you'll be losing and having to rehire about 30 people a year.

Skills for Care stats calculate that it costs £3,500 to replace a care worker accounting for all costs, but let's take a very modest estimate of £1,000 to replace a care worker for the purpose of this exercise.

Easy maths here – replacing 30 people a year will cost £30,000 a year.

With an induction plan in place like the one detailed in this chapter, you could save up to £15,000 by retaining those new hires that might have left. That's an enormous amount of money when you consider the small amount of work it takes to create a proper induction plan. Have we convinced you?

Induction processes may sit with yourself or you may be able to delegate this entire chapter to someone ready for some responsibility – see what they can do with the ideas listed here.

Induction vs orientation

Before we get started let's be clear on what induction is and how it's different from orientation. Orientation is generally what someone will do on their first day and will likely be paperwork, learning their way around the building and a little bit about how a typical day goes. Induction is a longer process, and normally would be a phase that lasts until the new hire passes their probation. That is often 3-6 months for most care companies.

We like to think of induction as the time it takes to get someone from 'newbie' to fully embedded member of the team. You want to do this in as quick a time as possible because it will save the company time and money, improve care quality and the quicker they get embedded, then the less they are likely to leave.

Have a think about the last time you were new in a company. What was important to you during those first days and weeks? What could have been done better by the company? Were you thrown in at the deep end with a 'sink or swim' attitude from your new employer? Sometimes, when we've been somewhere for a long time we forget what it feels like to be new. All of the tips in this chapter are designed to make a new hire feel valued and engaged from the start of their journey with you.

Tip 1 – The welcome letter

In this digital age the humble letter is often forgotten, but a welcome letter is the perfect way to create a great first impression to your new member of staff. Yes this could be digital, but there's something really nice about receiving a letter in the post and ideally you'd want to get this out to them a few days before they start.

Think back to the night before you started a new job. What were you nervous about? When we ask this question most people say: "What to wear" or "Will I make friends" or "What if I'm late on the first day". So, the idea is that the welcome letter addresses all of these, calms the nerves and really shows the new hire that you're looking forward to having them on board.

Some ideas for your welcome letter:

What to wear

Do you provide a uniform? Are trainers allowed? Are they likely to be going out and might need a waterproof jacket? Make it clear if you have a dress code and help them to feel comfortable in their choice of work attire for day one.

What to expect

Layout the timings for the day, let them know when to arrive and when they will finish. If there are roadworks near you or a school that causes a lot of traffic in the mornings, then make them aware. There is nothing worse than running late on your first day because of unexpected traffic!

The plan for day one

Will your new hire be doing mostly paperwork on the first day? Will they be meeting clients and getting stuck in straight away? Are you currently preparing for a CQC inspection that could happen on they day they start? Let them know who they are likely to meet on the first day and if you have a buddy system then let them know their name in the letter.

What to bring

Do you have lockers and should they bring a padlock? Is there a fridge if they want to bring a packed lunch? There's nothing worse than turning up on your first day with no cash or lunch and finding out that there's nothing close by to get something to eat. Why not assign someone to have lunch with them on their first day?

Anything else

Do you have a summer barbeque planned for that week? Someone's birthday? A visit from the mayor? Think of anything else that might be useful for them to know in advance. Again, you're showing them that they're included from the start.

Your values and culture

This is a great time to remind them of your values and include your culture or mission statement and any recent newsletters.

See our example welcome letter on the opposite page. This is something you could create a template for and easily tweak for each new hire. Imagine them receiving it and how they will feel to know you've gone to the effort to set them at ease before their first day. Imagine them showing it to their partner and the positive first impression their partner will have of your company. This stuff may sound simple, but it really makes a difference.

We've got a template of this welcome letter on the website: **www.careleadershandbook.co.uk** so feel free to download it from there and edit as you need.

MY CARE HOME
1 LONG ROAD
LONDON

To Sarah,

We are really looking forward to seeing you on 14th July for your first day here at My Care Home! Please arrive for 9am and Debbie will be waiting to show you around and get you settled.

Just to let you know there is a school at the end of the road and in the morning it can get quite busy with traffic so do allow yourself some extra time to get here, but there is free parking on the road behind us so you will be able to find somewhere to park easily.

On your first day we will take you through our policies and procedures in the morning and take you around to meet everyone. In the afternoon you might join some of the residents on a trip to the shops so wear trainers or comfy shoes and bring a coat.

Your buddy for the first week will be Chloe and she will have lunch with you on your first day. Feel free to bring a packed lunch as there is a fridge for staff, or there is a Tesco around the corner.

A date for your diary: We are having a family BBQ next Saturday 26th July and all staff, residents and families are invited. We do this every year and it's always good fun if you're able to attend. Children and dogs are also very welcome!

If you've got any questions before your first day please give us a call and I've included a copy of our values and culture statements to give you an idea of what it's like here at My Care Home.

See you on Monday,

Dawn Smith

Tip 2 – Training

No doubt there will be various training courses and workshops that your new hire will need to complete as they progress through their induction. Some will be the same for every new hire, so why not create a checklist with every bit of training, including any computer systems training, health and safety, compliance, care certificates, anything you can think of! Give that checklist along with ideal completion dates to your new hire on their first day for them to keep hold of.

By doing this it gives them easy goals, along with an understanding of what is expected of them and by when. They can keep track of their own progress and take responsibility for making sure they receive the training they need.

This also helps to promote a culture of learning and self-leadership within the company which is good to embed from the start.

Tip 3 – Career progression

You may have spoken about career progression during the interview process, but after your new hire has started it's time to wipe the slate clean and have the conversation again. They may have been nervous in the interview and said what they thought they wanted you to hear, so it's good to start from scratch and do this very early on. Why? Your new hire might have their eye on another job that they think offers what they want. You don't want someone jumping ship just because you didn't have a conversation.

The best way to do this is make it a relaxed chat about how they're getting on and learn more about them as a person. Are they interested in progressing in the company or happy as they are? Quite often we make the mistake of thinking people want to progress when they might have no desire and that's ok – we need people to make up the core workforce and need to respect them for that.

If they do express a desire to progress, then ask them about where they'd like to see themselves in the next year and a few years' time. Help them to understand likely timescales and name someone in the company who has progressed in the way that your new hire wants to. Try to get them together for a chat so that your new hire can really have a good picture painted to them of their potential career journey from the person who's already done it. It's a powerful way of getting them bought into the company and focused on their goals.

Tip 4 – Social inclusion

This is often the most important factor for anyone starting a new job and people often say the best thing about their job is 'the people' so it's important to really consider how good your team are at embracing new hires and embedding them as one of the team.

If you have a buddy or mentor system, then think about the people who are looking after the new members of the team. Are they the best possible ambassador for your business? What do you think they would say about the company behind closed doors?

You want to find a champion - a naturally curious and enthusiastic person who can be put in charge of looking out for new hires, and that way their positive attitude will likely rub off onto the new employee. Make sure the new hire has someone to have lunch with on their first day and someone to make them a cup of tea in their break - these small efforts go a long way.

Tip 5 - Feedback

The best person to give you feedback on your induction process is your new hire while they are going through it! Make time within their induction to ask them how their induction is going and what could be improved. This is their chance to be open and honest and let you know about any gaps or anything additional that would help. It's also a good time to find out what they've observed about the company, the culture and the way you operate. Do they have any ideas from a previous employer that could work well?

By encouraging their feedback you're showing that as a company you value their opinion and that you support an open culture. It also gives you the opportunity to make changes, if necessary, for the next new hire going through induction.

Tip 6 – Ensure your values are aligned

If you've followed other steps within this book, the values of your new hire should already align with those of the company. Hopefully this will have come across during the recruitment process and they will have been reminded of the values in their welcome letter. Make sure this also carries through into their induction. Are they seeing people in the team embody the values and recognition for the people that do?

If you can capture what it means to embody the values of your organisation in the early days with your new hire, then they're going to have an emotional connection with the company, and studies show that people who have an emotional connection are far more likely to go the extra mile.

Induction may be part of a bigger project in developing your company culture, but don't forget those that are new who can often be moulded more easily to embody the values you want.

So, there you have it. Five tips that may take a short amount of time to get set up, but can be easily replicated for each new hire. Why don't you involve someone in the creation of the welcome letter and writing up the process for induction to give them some additional responsibility? If they read this chapter then they will get a good feel for what's required and may even have some ideas you can incorporate.

Hiring and interview

We're going to take a step back now to the hiring process and this won't be a long chapter but it is something we want to cover.

We are often first introduced to a care company to support the hiring process and the typical comments we hear are: "We struggle to recruit staff", "They leave within a few weeks of hiring" and "They seemed fantastic in the interview... what went wrong?!"

Many care companies feel like they are on a continual cycle of hiring due to staff turnover issues, so hopefully this entire section of the book on developing culture will begin to have a positive impact on staff retention but appreciate that change doesn't happen overnight.

For tips on finding people in the first place we recommend Neil Eastwood's book; Saving Social Care, and if you've ever caught him speaking at an event you'll know that he shares some great tips on how to find care staff and make the most of referral schemes.

In this chapter we are going to look at the interview process, share some tips when interviewing and also, some common mistakes that we see.

Cautions during the hiring process

Whether you're a large care company or a small one, you probably use the selection practices below and it's important to bear in mind that most of these look backwards or are performed under controlled conditions:

- CV – is self written
- References – may not always reflect the truth
- Agencies – will always show candidates in a good light – they have their own agenda!
- Probation period – will involve supervision and a controlled environment

It's worth bearing in mind that besides someone choosing to leave of their own accord, the reason why people succeed in an interview, only to fail later is often because they are able to hide many of the things that make them a 'risky hire' during the interview process.

There is a move towards values-based recruitment in care, and it can certainly highlight people who have the strengths needed to work in care such as empathy and engagement, being able to follow directions and having good intuition.

Think about areas that people are able to hide during interview though. Overwhelm, stress (whether personal or at work), tolerance and compassion, high performance frustrations which we looked at in the first section of the book.

If we take tolerance as an example, it can easily be displayed, but we know from some of the Panorama documentaries of recent times that it's possible to have people working in care who actually don't have tolerance and this can be a big risk to a care company, in terms of client safety and also the company brand.

Consider what scenario-based questions you can ask to uncover potential red flags. Ask about their current role and responsibilities to try to determine if the role you are offering would be more challenging. Ask what frustrates them in their current job. What do they enjoy doing? How do they recharge outside of work? What bores them about their current role? How have they dealt with stressful scenarios both inside and outside of work in the past? These types of questions will help you to get more out of the person than the standard interview questions they are used to being asked.

A more robust interview process

Be cautious when interviewing of choosing people based on their personality. Personality is proven to be a very poor indicator of how someone is likely to perform at work. We also see managers fall into the habit of hiring a 'mini-me', which can result in a team with little diversity and gaps in skills.

Whilst gut instinct can count for a lot while interviewing, be aware of something called confirmation bias.

An example of confirmation bias could be that someone who applies for a job is qualified and prepared to work nights. If this is a position you struggle to recruit for you could miss any red flags because you're already wanting that person to be successful in the interview.

Other biases can be around judging superficial factors such as tattoos or even intuition bias, particularly if you're under a lot of stress yourself as that is when your own intuition could be weaker.

Be aware that someone who comes across very shy in an interview could be a superstar care professional, but not have experience being interviewed so it actually relies on your talent as an interviewer to tease out the star qualities in them. Someone who gives all the right answers to the questions could have worked for many different care companies, so they might have the experience but there may also be a reason why they've worked in so many places! Bear in mind that the majority of people (around 60% or more) will have worked for another care company before, so they will have already been through the interview process at least once.

Try bringing someone else into the interview to help you to be more objective. This could be another member of staff or even a client. You'll get a great feel for how the interviewee will behave with clients and a walk around the premises to meet some of them will also reveal a lot.

Be sure to emphasise the values, any mission statement or culture statements and create questions that will help uncover whether this person aligns with those values. Skills can be taught, but if their values don't align with the company then they may not be the right fit.

If you're looking to take your values-based recruitment even further then it may be worth considering using an assessment as part of the hiring process, which can support a more objective recruitment process and help standardise interviewing across multiple locations. To learn more about the Judgement Index assessment, which measures values-based behaviours, see the pages at the end of the book.

Wellbeing in care

Our final chapter is focused on how to improve the wellbeing of your team. We are sure that if you've followed the book and started the process of completing the various exercises then there will already be a lift in the wellbeing of the team, but it's such an important part of company culture that often gets overlooked so we want to make sure we cover it fully and give you some final tips and ideas to set you on your way.

> **Richard Branson said:** *"Clients do not come first. Employees come first. If you take care of your employees, they will take care of the clients."*

If you can look after the wellbeing of your staff, then they will do the job of looking after your clients. This is important to remember, because often the whole focus of a care company is solely on the clients and the staff are missed.

To highlight this, we wanted to share some research from NACAS; the National Association of Care and Support Workers on wellbeing in care. It was conducted by Care Research in 2018 and found:

- The current staff turnover rate in social care is 30.7%.
- 24% of care staff intend to leave the sector altogether within five years.
- 61% of care staff believe that their work has had a negative impact on their mental health.

This is only a small snapshot of the results but with some positive action we believe these statistics could improve.

What's the true cost of poor staff wellbeing?

We often think of wellbeing as something that can't be quantified or drilled down to a monetary cost on the business...

- But if you add your current staff turnover...
- With the current cost of staff absence and agency fees...
- With poor quality of work because people aren't happy...
- And the impact on the culture as a result of this...

According to Skills For Care the average cost to replace a care professional is £3,500. Add that to staff absence, and did you know that unhappy employees take on average an extra 15 sick days per year? Can you think of one person on your team who might be doing that? It's not just about what it costs in money but how it then impacts across the company.

We see a lot of care budgets that go to health and safety, audits, training, risk management and we appreciate that these are mandatory and easily measured. Perhaps there's some confusion around how to support staff wellbeing or a misconception that it needs to cost a lot of money? We speak to companies who think the way to improve wellbeing of staff is to incentivise them with rewards (if they can afford to) but remember the chapter early on in the book that discussed extrinsic pleasure and how it is a short-term solution? Yes, a gift voucher or treat will get people excited for a short time, but there's a better way of tapping into those intrinsic pleasures which will drive positive wellbeing for the long term.

What makes up workplace wellbeing?

It's good to clarify wellbeing and what it means in the workplace, because that can help you put a plan together to improve it. Wellbeing and workplace wellbeing can have different definitions, but a piece of research by a company called A Great Place To Work identified four main areas that defined workplace wellbeing, and we think they fit well within the care sector.

Workplace wellbeing is driven by four things:

Values aligned behaviour

As a care professional, you want to know that the company you work for is on the same mission that you are. Are your values aligned? Have you ever had to do something for a company you worked for that didn't align with your values?

We hear this the most about 15-minute visits in home care. Whilst the company may have a contract to conduct 15-minute visits, quite often the care professionals feel some internal turmoil about not being able to give enough time for clients. Over time this may cause the person to look for a company that conducts longer visits so that it fits with their values about care delivery.

We've covered values and how to develop them in a lot of detail so far in the book. If you've created culture statements with your team then you will already be developing values-aligned behaviour. But this does highlight how important it is to put effort into the values in order to improve wellbeing.

Teamwork

Is everyone in it together? Do they support each other? Or do people say: "Oh no, that's not my job. I'll do mine and you do yours"

We spend most of our life at work and we want to get on with those we work with. Consider whether you have any cliques within your team that could make new staff feel unwelcome or other members of the team feel isolated. Teamwork is a real key factor in workplace wellbeing and anything you can do to drive the feeling that you're in it together and supporting each other can really impact.

Processes

This might seem like a strange one at first, but it's about having the tools and resources to do the job properly and clear processes in place so that staff are not stressed or frustrated when trying to do their work. Do you make it easy for them to get on with it or are systems failing which can cause stress?

You may understand the pain of this one yourself. If you've ever had computer issues or long-winded paperwork processes, then you'll know they can really drag morale down and get in the way of work. It's interesting how they can also impact on wellbeing and some simple reviews of how job applications work or the care planning systems can make a positive difference in a company.

Recognition

We've covered this in detail in previous chapters. Are you recognising your team for the great work they are doing? We often find that people working in care get on with the job and don't think they are doing anything special, but are they reminded that in fact, they are? Do they get a thank you?

Recognition is so easy to weave into a company without costing anything, and as a start we recommend celebrating Professional Care Workers Day on 4th September every year. See the website: **www.nacas.org.uk** for ideas on how to get involved.

Even though we've covered these areas within the book, it's useful to keep these 4 pillars of workplace wellbeing in your mind when you're developing the culture. Perhaps print the image and have it somewhere to remind you to ask yourself and your team: "Are we driving a culture of wellbeing here?"

WHAT DRIVES WELLBEING?

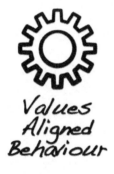

Values
Aligned
Behaviour

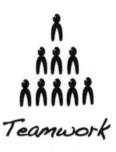

Teamwork

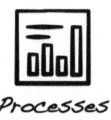

Processes

Recognition

Create and promote a wellbeing policy within the company

A simple way to begin the drive to a wellbeing culture is to create a wellbeing policy that can be shared with staff, clients, families, included within a staff handbook and logged in your CQC evidence.

Remember that company values tend to be about the clients, but a wellbeing policy can be more of a mission statement for the people who work for you. Think about how powerful that could be when it comes to hiring. A wellbeing policy or mission statement for staff will set you aside from competition as it is something care professionals might have never seen before.

We've created a wellbeing policy template which can be downloaded and then edited from the website: **www.careleadershandbook.co.uk**. We recommend using it as a guide, as the best way to create one is to involve the team.

The wellbeing policy really picks up from the work you will have done developing culture statements, and they may even translate directly into your policy. Make sure the policy covers what it really means to support and promote wellbeing in your company.

Here are some questions that may give some ideas of what to include:

- Are people given the day off on their birthday?
- Do you have a relaxing space for staff?
- Can people take time to eat lunch?
- Is thank you part of your culture?
- Do you support staff to achieve their goals?

Another way to get ideas on how to support wellbeing is to look for books, articles and newsletters that aren't just from care-related companies. Take inspiration from outside of the sector as you can get some great unusual ideas.

Once you've created the wellbeing policy and distributed it to staff then make sure you also share it across your social media channels, create a notice board within the company to share it to visitors, and maybe even contact the local newspaper about it! It's bound to attract positive attention, from both potential clients and potential staff.

Other simple wellbeing strategies

Create a zen den

> **Sophie says:** *"I walk into care companies and find the only place for peace and quiet is a smoking shed – which is not very wellbeing orientated!"*

Are there any spaces dedicated just for staff? Somewhere where they can take a proper break without being disturbed?

Try to create a relaxing space, perhaps with books and magazines, a pinboard to share positive quotes, stories and things people might take an interest in outside of work such as local Zumba classes.

The order of the elephant

We've borrowed this idea from a book called The Happiness Advantage by Shaun Achor, and if you like the idea then it's worth reading the entire book.

In it, Shaun shares a story about a Danish company who bought a big cuddly elephant and it was for any employee to give to another as reward for doing something exemplary.

The key to the exercise is that it wasn't for management to decide who deserved the elephant, the decision lay within the team. That employee would then take possession of the elephant and the company found that many people would stop and ask about it, which encouraged the employee to share how they came to have it.

We think this idea could fit well into a care environment. An elephant might not be the most practical way to recreate it, but what about a badge or sash?

It's a great way to encourage peer to peer recognition and positive story telling.

Communication via mobile

Many care companies now operate a WhatsApp group for people to communicate with, and it's a step in the right direction as most people have mobile phones and access them regularly.

So, we might sound like we are contradicting ourselves now because we don't think care companies should be using a WhatsApp group as a best way of encouraging communication.

Why?

Most people use WhatsApp for personal use, to keep in touch with friends and family, and so when work messages start appearing in personal time they can be invasive and cause stress and anxiety. Even if someone chooses to ignore work messages when they're not at work, seeing them can play on their mind and so it's not the best tool if you're trying to drive a culture of wellbeing.

There is a better solution in the form of another free app called Slack. Slack works in a similar way to WhatsApp but it was created specifically for work use which makes it easy to separate from your personal life and even turn off notifications or set 'away' times. As well as having different groups or teams within Slack you can also have different topics or threads for team meeting ideas, shifts, evidence capture and CQC updates which means communication is easy to follow.

If your team already use WhatsApp then it should be easy to switch to Slack, and we've had many care teams tell us it's worked really well for them.

Revamp your job titles

What would your clients call your job title if they described it by the impact you have on their lives?

This is such a good way of starting a conversation about what job titles should be. We've heard many people say that the term 'care worker' doesn't cut it anymore and that's caused them to give their job titles a refresh. Do you think that could promote a feeling of positivity in your company? Many are changing to the title 'care professional' because it's a professional career and should be seen as such. The same could also be said of client titles and we've seen many move away from the term 'service user' to something more personal.

Play positive Tetris

Our last tip is difficult to describe and is more of a behavioural change but could make a real difference to the wellbeing of the team.

Do you know what Tetris is? Just in case you don't, it's an old computer game played on a Game Boy. The aim is to stack different shaped blocks in an order, so they fit together. For a piece of research conducted in Harvard people had to play Tetris for a few hours a day. The unexpected side-effect was that the people started to see Tetris shapes everywhere they went.

How does this relate to care?

In care there is an ingrained habit to focus on the negative. Your job is spot things that are wrong with a client, any potential risk, potential safeguarding incidents. Managing compliance and mitigating risk is a crucial aspect of the care sector. The side-effect of this is that it builds a habit of spotting what's wrong instead of what's right. This habit will be even further ingrained in compliance managers!

Negativity is infectious and can spread through an organisation like second-hand smoke. By playing positive Tetris during the course of the day - trying to spot the good things that are happening and encourage others to do the same, you can help to change any negative habits that have formed. You might begin by simply ending every team meeting with gratitude or recognition. Try to make the last thing you do before you leave for the day something that spreads positivity.

Before long people will start to absorb your behaviour and spotting and recognising the positive will become a natural habit within the company.

Now you have four pillars of workplace wellbeing to think about, a wellbeing policy to write with your team and some strategies to put in place to lift the overall wellbeing. We are sure that once these things are in place the impact throughout the entire company will be felt – not just by the staff but by your clients as well. Keep in mind the Richard Branson quote, he knows his stuff!

Summary

We really hope you have enjoyed the journey through the book with us and you should now be well on your way to leading your culture, your team and of course yourself to success.

Change doesn't happen overnight. We called this book a handbook for a reason – it should be a resource that you refer back to again and again. Make sure you head to the website **www.careleadershandbook.co.uk** to print off all the templates shared in the book and start to incorporate them into your supervisions and appraisals.

The password to access the page is: **judgement**

Don't be afraid to practice, make mistakes and keep trying until you feel it's starting to make a difference. Remember that this sector needs more self-leaders, and we have no doubt you will already be influencing those around you to more positive outcomes.

Feel free to reach out for advice or for further information about our leadership academies and the Judgement Index, we will always be delighted to share and help where possible.

Good luck on your journey,

Sophie and Rob

The Judgement Index Assessment

The Judgement Index is an online assessment that measures values-based behaviours and is used by care companies across the UK to support hiring, development and leadership.

Our Care Sector report has been benchmarked against high performing care workers and has enabled us to create a concise, easy to use report that comes with interview questions to help guide the conversation.

As the assessment only takes around fifteen minutes to complete, and reports are instantly generated, it is a popular choice for care companies looking to identify the right people for the job, particularly when they struggle with staff turnover. The Judgement Index allows interviewers to be more objective and helps to standardise recruitment practices across multiple managers and locations.

By using the Judgement Index assessment with existing staff members, we are able to produce team reports which can highlight collective development areas, enabling you to target your training more effectively. You will also see who in your team match the qualities of successful leaders in care and who is more likely to be a compliance risk meaning you can focus your management efforts where they are needed.

The Care Sector Report is also an incredibly useful tool during the appraisal process, as it allows a more meaningful conversation around strengths and development areas. Our clients are trained to pick out key areas of the report to discuss during appraisals and set actionable goals which can be measured the following year.

Our case studies show dramatic reductions in staff turnover as well as improvements in staff, both personally and professionally when the Judgement Index is utilised throughout the company.

If you'd like to know more about using the Judgement Index in your company, then get in touch or see more on the website: **www.judgementindex.co.uk**

Our Leadership Academies

Our popular leadership academies were the inspiration for this book! If you've found the book useful and would like to take things further, then an academy or workshop is a great next step.

Our Leadership Academies and workshops range from half a day up to a ten-day leadership course and we have over 20+ modules which can be adapted for your team's needs. We've run them for private companies, councils and care associations for people at all different levels in care.

Our training is interactive, practical, challenging but fun! We aim to deliver leadership techniques and models that the delegates can go back and put into practice immediately in their care environment.

We hope the book has given you some great ideas, but there's nothing like learning in real life, so get in touch if you'd like a brochure and more information.

Email: **gabby@judgementindex.co.uk** for a brochure and see the website: **www.judgementindex.co.uk** for more, including a video of one of our academy's highlights.

We will leave the final word to one of our clients:

> *"From a business point of view, we now have confident leaders who are showing and leading the way, enthusiastic and passionate in what they do, confident in being able to voice and demonstrate new ideas and ways of working. They have team meetings, mottos have appeared all over the units reminding staff and every one why we are here.*
>
> *Relatives have commented on the difference in the participants behaviours and how much more confident they are.*
>
> *I now have more staff wanting to become the new set of Marches Care Academy Leaders."* **Carey Bloomer, managing director, Marches Care**

Printed in Great Britain
by Amazon

39956554R00112